Praise for *The Mommy Docs' Ultimate Guide to Pregnancy and Birth*

"Throughout, the authors deliver practical tips and emotional support for coping with both complicated and uncomplicated pregnancies as well as the things that can go wrong, such as miscarriages or infertility. A great resource for anyone seeking information on pregnancy, childbirth, and the first weeks after birth."
—*Library Journal*

"Comprehensive and engaging." —*Kirkus Reviews*

"Written in an easy to understand way . . . Every woman who is pregnant or wishing to get pregnant will find this book a great resource." —*Portland Book Review*

"A comprehensive guide to pretty much everything that happens from preparing for pregnancy through the 'fourth trimester' after birth." —*Deseret News*

"What could be better than a guide to pregnancy and birth written by doctors who are also moms? . . . [A] comprehensive new book . . . Written in a clear and friendly style. Packed with real-life stories from new moms and tested practical tips, this extraordinary guide is a reassuring resource for a healthy and stress-free pregnancy." —*Tucson Citizen*

"Full of . . . useful tidbits . . . With common-sense information and advice on everything from breastfeeding to baby blues, these are the doctors every new mommy wants at her side. The comparisons to the seminal *What to Expect When You're Expecting* are inevitable, but the Mommy Docs write in a more conversational, matter-of-fact tone . . . A thorough and useful guide from conception to pregnancy and delivery." —*BookPage*

"So filled with medically sound advice, intelligently presented case histories, extensive debunking of myths, and all-around sensible writing, that the book itself becomes a thing you might not expect while expecting: a super-clear, super-helpful, easy-to-read and easy-to-use guide that beautifully balances the medical with the personal." —InfoDad.com

"It's the Mommy Docs' comforting tone that makes this guide both invaluable and appealing. Recognizing that pregnancy is as much about emotional changes as it is about physical changes, they set their guide apart from others by providing heartfelt personal experiences and those of many of their patients. Whether it's a reader's first, second, or even third child, there's good advice for every kind of pregnant mother." —*Foreword*

YOUR PREGNANCY,
YOUR WAY

Also by Allison Hill, MD

The Mommy Docs' Ultimate Guide to Pregnancy and Birth
with Yvonne Bohn, MD and Alane Park, MD

YOUR PREGNANCY, YOUR WAY

Everything You Need to Know about Natural Pregnancy and Childbirth

Allison Hill, MD

with Sheila Curry Oakes

Da Capo
∞
LIFE
LONG

DESIGNED BY LINDA MARK
Set in 12 point Warnock Pro Light by Perseus Books

Cataloging-in-Publication data for this book is available from the Library of Congress.

First Da Capo Press edition 2017
ISBN: 978-0-7382-1910-3 (paperback)
ISBN: 978-0-7382-1911-0 (e-book)

Published by Da Capo Press, an imprint of Perseus Books, LLC, a subsidiary of Hachette Book Group, Inc.
www.dacapopress.com

Note: The information in this book is true and complete to the best of our knowledge. This book is intended only as an informative guide for those wishing to know more about health issues. In no way is this book intended to replace, countermand, or conflict with the advice given to you by your own physician. The ultimate decision concerning care should be made between you and your doctor. We strongly recommend you follow his or her advice. Information in this book is general and is offered with no guarantees on the part of the authors or Da Capo Press. The authors and publisher disclaim all liability in connection with the use of this book. The names and identifying details of people associated with events described in this book have been changed. Any similarity to actual persons is coincidental.

Da Capo Press books are available at special discounts for bulk purchases in the U.S. by corporations, institutions, and other organizations. For more information, please contact the Special Markets Department at Perseus Books, 2300 Chestnut Street, Suite 200, Philadelphia, PA 19103, or call (800) 810-4145, ext. 5000, or e-mail special.markets@perseusbooks.com.

10 9 8 7 6 5 4 3 2 1

To the mothers who have the courage to insist on a natural and mindful birth experience, and to the doctors and midwives who are dedicated to providing care in a safe and respectful way.

CONTENTS

A NOTE ON PRONOUNS

FOR CONVENIENCE, I OFTEN USE A SINGLE PRONOUN—*HE* OR *SHE*—to refer to a health-care professional, spouse, or partner; or I may refer to a father or husband rather than a wife, co-parent, or co-mother. I have attempted to alternate use of these pronouns and titles throughout the book. I do not in any case mean to imply that professionals or partners are exclusively one gender or another.

ACKNOWLEDGMENTS

I WOULD LIKE TO THANK THE THOUSANDS OF PATIENTS WHO HAVE chosen me as their doctor over the last twenty years. You have shared the most intimate moments of your life with me, and for that, I am forever grateful.

I was honored to write this book with Sheila Curry Oakes. Sheila brought an enthusiasm to the project that gave my words life. Her fresh perspective and patience were greatly welcomed.

I appreciate the hard work of my editors Renée Sedliar and Lisa Kaufman, project editor Amber Morris, and copyeditor Iris Bass. I'd also like to thank marketing director Kevin Hanover, publicity director Lissa Warren, and publisher John Radziewicz at Da Capo Press. Thank you for believing in me and finding the book inside me.

I owe gratitude to Andrea Harrow, the librarian at Good Samaritan Hospital, for her contribution in locating the hundreds of research studies that I reference in this book. Andrea was available on a moment's notice to find what I needed, even from obscure obstetrical journals. Her support and encouragement won't be forgotten.

I would like to thank my family—my parents, Pat and Bob; and my children, Luke and Kat—for their support and inspiration.

Thanks to Anita and Myron, for their advice, generosity, and kindness.

And finally, deepest thanks to my love, Eric, who has encouraged me to think outside the box and believed in me unconditionally.

This book would not be possible without all of you.

INTRODUCTION

I N MY TWENTY-YEAR CAREER AS AN OB-GYN, I'VE DELIVERED THOU-
sands of babies and have seen every type of birth. A mother relaxing in a warm bath, breathing deeply with her contractions. A
woman being wheeled down the halls of the hospital for an emergency cesarean as blood pours from her placenta previa. A woman
who has an epidural, listening to music and talking excitedly with
her family about the future. Each scene is different, but as the top of
a baby's head emerges, I can feel my own heart racing in my chest.
I love to steal a glance at the faces of the family as they see their son
or daughter for the first time. More important, I can breathe a sigh
of relief that the baby is safe.

But what type of birth is best? Some would argue that having
your baby at home, surrounded by supportive family and friends,
and with minimal medical intervention, is the way it should be done.
Others view childbirth as risky and would only want to have a baby
in a hospital where a doctor, anesthesiologist, and all of the current
technology are available. There are arguments to be made on each
side of this debate, and I don't think there will ever be a clear con-
sensus. I believe that the focus shouldn't be on what "type" of birth
is best but, rather, on how to achieve the safest, most personalized,
respectful care in all possible settings.

I was anxious during my own pregnancy and I'm an obstetrician! I believed everything that really mattered was almost sure to go right. But I also knew that things could go wrong. Although my delivery didn't go exactly as planned, luckily, my own OB and I had agreed about how to make my pregnancy as safe as possible while achieving my vision for the birth, even if that meant making choices that would differ from the way most doctors would handle things. I had the inside track. That's not the way it works for everyone.

It may seem surprising that obstetricians don't always make decisions purely on the basis of the most up-to-date medical practice and what is best for the patient. Our patients have a right to that kind of care. They should feel that their doctor is *on* their side, not just *at* their side. But the truth is, sometimes we make decisions based on other concerns, such as the threat of malpractice lawsuits, our own preferences and training, hospital policies, and personal convenience. The good news is that you, as a mother-to-be, can enable your obstetrician to provide the best care by working together in a way that your doctor will welcome.

This book is my opportunity to reflect candidly on what I have learned as a busy obstetrician and to explore the unspoken facets of this field. What I have written may be considered controversial. I'm here to tell you that much of the advice you hear from friends, pregnancy websites, and even doctors isn't based on scientific evidence. Numerous conventional medical practices need to change—and we know it. Why then, do we stick to an outdated way of doing things, disseminating unfounded advice? To put it simply: because that's the way things have always been done.

I will explain the basis of medical decision-making and how to empower yourself to work side by side with your doctor or midwife on this journey. This book will help you understand the birth process so you may have realistic expectations for what may happen, and what is and is not in your control. The more clearly you understand what you want, and the better you are able to adapt to whatever comes your way, the better your birth experience will be.

New mothers and their babies are best off if the mother is happy and confident. The pregnancy goes more smoothly and any problems that come up seem less worrisome. Even the mother's relationship with her baby gets off to a better start when she has a positive birth experience. But the definition of a positive experience varies greatly from woman to woman. I have seen some mothers who know exactly what they want from the beginning and are able to achieve all of their goals. Others were able to adjust their expectations and have a satisfying experience despite their birth plan's being altered at every step along the way. Unfortunately, still others are needlessly disappointed in themselves and their birth because things didn't go as planned and they had an epidural or required a cesarean.

I don't want to give the impression that you can pick exactly how you want your birth to be, and that it will follow that script. Medical issues may arise for you or your baby that make it impossible, or once you are in labor you may simply not want to do it. But as you plan for a natural pregnancy and birth, this book will help you navigate through any unforeseen complications that come your way, so that you may stay as close as possible to your original vision. Your birth can be on your terms, feeling that you are part of the team and that your goals are respected. I hope that what you read here will empower you to be successful, however you bring your baby into the world.

Instead of focusing on the small details of how their baby came into the world, my patients who have enjoyed their births the most have shifted their focus to the final, positive outcome, learned to see the big picture, avoided rigid judgment from others, and eased up on the perfectionism. The ability to remain flexible and let go of what "should" happen will serve as a great asset during the many years of motherhood and childrearing to come. Natural pregnancy and childbirth is a wonderful choice but might not be right for you. Whether or not you stick to your original plan, have multiple interventions or none at all, doesn't determine whether you are a good mother. At your child's birth, your journey as a mother is just beginning.

WHAT DOES A "NATURAL" BIRTH MEAN, ANYWAY?

WOMEN HAVE BEEN GIVING BIRTH FOR CENTURIES; WHAT CAN BE more natural than that? Well, it is not quite so simple. For each and every woman, *natural* means something different. The definition depends on where you live, the customs in your family, and, most important, whether you view pregnancy as inherently safe or inherently risky.

In recent times, the word *natural* is often used to characterize things we assume to be healthier, safer, and better for us. For some women, having a natural birth simply means that they want to deliver vaginally instead of by cesarean section. To others, it means not using pain medication, although an IV and fetal monitoring are welcome. Some believe that all births are natural as long as what is done is best for the mom and the baby. Others think *natural* implies avoiding the hospital altogether and trusting their body to give birth the way women have done for generations, delivering in the familiar setting of their own home or in a peaceful birthing center without beeping machines and rushed medical personnel.

───── **HOW MY PATIENTS DEFINE NATURAL CHILDBIRTH** ─────

- "Not using pain medication."
- "Delivering vaginally."
- "Minimizing medical intervention."
- "Choosing pain."
- "Having an un-medicated birth."
- "Bringing a baby into the world alive."
- "Having control over my delivery."
- "Trusting my body to give birth the way it was meant to."
- "Having a baby the way I want."

Calling a birth "natural" brings up the question of what would constitute an "unnatural" birth. For those of us in the medical field, the opposite of a natural birth is one with interventions. Yet, in lay terms, to say that a birth is not "natural" implies that the event is not as good, or even harmful. Is a birth experience artificial or abnormal when medical interventions are chosen, or become necessary?

Influences on Our View of Childbirth

Thanks to Hollywood, when most of us picture labor, we think of a woman on her back in a hospital bed, surrounded by machines, screaming and sweating, perhaps yelling a string of curse words as she bears down with each contraction. The father-to-be grips her hand, white-faced and helpless, feeling faint. A tense nurse shouts instructions as a doctor catches the baby's emerging head. Labor is fast, furious, and intense.

We almost never see labor depicted as a relaxed, peaceful experience. Watching the process play out in its slow, methodical way, sometimes lasting for days, wouldn't make for a dramatic moment in a movie. It is no surprise that many women approach labor fearfully, focusing on the pain, rather than anticipating it as the extraordinary event it can be.

Our view of pregnancy and childbirth is also influenced by the experiences of women who have gone before us—the well-meaning family and friends who, with good intentions, want to prepare us for the worst, and explain the labor process in frightening detail. Women freely discuss their emergency cesareans and the unforeseen twists and turns, and all of it seems commonplace. As "survivors," they feel obligated to share their words of wisdom. Even if their stories are reassuring, the birth you want, or that will be best for you and your baby, may not be the same as your friend's, sister's, or mother's. Unfortunately, you may hear more negatives than positives. A woman with an unfavorable birth experience will frequently share her horror story with anyone who will listen, whereas a woman with a positive experience will hold the memory privately with just a few friends and family.

the doctor's diary

When I meet a woman for the first time and tell her I'm an obstetrician, I almost always hear her birth story. Nearly every description includes details of something that went wrong or was unexpected. I'm pleasantly surprised if she tells me how beautiful her birth was. Even the story of our own birth as relayed by our mother unknowingly shapes our views of labor. Inevitably, you will share your story someday—with friends, colleagues, and your own daughter. Consider how your description will influence her perspective about childbirth in the future.

The shared experience of pregnancy should bond women together and encourage them to be supportive of one another at this important time. Finding a group of women who share your views and beliefs can be invaluable. Childbirth is not a competition in which prizes are awarded to the mother who was able to give birth without an epidural or who pushed out the biggest baby. Sometimes, you may feel that any decision you make about your pregnancy can lead to a conversation loaded with judgment. Are you going to have a natural birth? Will you use an epidural? How long are you planning to breastfeed? No matter how you answer, or how well thought-out your decision, someone, somewhere, will tell you that you're doing it wrong. Remember, your choices are ultimately between you, your partner, and your provider. Identify a few close friends to confide in, who want the best for you and will support you in your decisions.

Childbirth from the Home to the Hospital

Until the 1900s, childbirth took place in the home. Women commonly labored in an area that was closed off from the rest of the house, surrounded by female family members and friends. They used herbs and drank caudle, a spiced wine, for pain relief and relaxation. As active labor got under way, they were kept warm with the windows closed and candles burning in the room. Once the baby was born, they would remain in this room for a month, being attended by their families. Despite the comfortable environment, childbirth was regarded as dangerous because, in those days, many women did not survive. In the United States, prior to 1900, 1 in 1,000 women and 40 in 1,000 babies died during birth.

In 1531, an innovative military surgeon, Dr. Ambroise Paré, started a school for midwives in Paris. One of his pupil's wives, Louise Bourgeois, became a well-known midwife to the royal court of France, and in 1609, published an influential book on how to practice the craft. She promoted the idea of letting nature take its course: "The time of the birth having arrived, they [midwives] did what their art demanded, which was, the child coming nicely, to reassure friends and family, keep her in a good position, have her eat as appropriate, keep her moderately warm, then help her to use her labor pains to bring everything to a happy conclusion."[1]

In the late-1800s, there was a shift in philosophy about childbirth as more men became trained in obstetrics. It wasn't just a field for midwives who had learned their skills as apprentices; it was a science that attracted surgeons. "Lying-in" hospitals were founded in urban areas, and women would travel there to have their babies delivered by male midwives, or *accoucheurs*. Birth became separate from family life. The use of lifesaving antibiotics and antiseptic solutions became more common. Pain medication was available, and cesareans were a viable option.

Dr. Joseph DeLee, who founded the Chicago Lying-In Hospital in 1899, is considered the father of modern obstetrics. Because of the high complication rates in childbirth, he wondered "if nature did not intend for women to be used up in the process of reproduction, in a manner analogous to salmon, which die after spawning." He believed that labor should be actively managed so as to protect the life of the mother and baby. He suggested that a laboring woman should be heavily sedated to the point of being unconscious, to allow the cervix to dilate. A generous episiotomy should be made and the baby pulled out with forceps. Birth became a completely passive process and family members were not involved.

Dr. DeLee's philosophy influenced generations of obstetricians. By the 1950s, 90 percent of babies in the United States were born in hospitals, and 70 percent of those were delivered with forceps. Hospital staff performed the duties previously delegated to family members. Most women were sedated with ether, giving birth in beds that had rails like a crib and wearing helmets so they wouldn't injure themselves while they were medicated. As technology advanced, medical interventions, such as electronic fetal monitoring, ultrasounds, and epidurals, became the norm.

Today, doctors have replaced midwives, now attending 92 percent of births in the United States. Cesarean sections account for 33 percent of births. Instead of expecting something to go wrong, many women assume that the advantages of modern medicine will guarantee a perfect outcome. They want the latest technology to be available and to have the option to deliver their baby pain-free.

Natural Versus Medicated: The Debate

Women want their birth to be safe. But what *safety* means is open to discussion. Should you receive medication to speed up the labor or to reduce its pain? Is it better to let nature take its course or undergo an intervention that has its own risks? In the debate over natural or medicated, is there a right answer? The controversy can turn as heated as a political argument! People on both sides of this issue firmly believe that they are doing what is best for themselves and their babies.

Medications to prevent infections, drugs to reduce bleeding, cesareans—these advances in medicine have saved the life of numerous mothers and babies. However, interventions have become the norm, even in low-risk pregnancies. Some of these have undoubtedly benefited families. Others have little evidence to support their use, and a few may actually be harmful. These days, finding the balance between the natural experience and medical interventions is particularly challenging.

Natural childbirth advocates believe that using interventions during labor diminishes the birthing experience, puts women at increased risk, and may have long-term consequences for both mother and baby. They see the pain of labor as "good" and even necessary. Medical interventions are viewed as dangerous and overused, and employed for the convenience of the doctor. They believe that the more we know about pregnancy and birth, the more we lose sight of how perfectly designed it is. They feel safer away from a hospital than in one. They contend that women who have a natural childbirth recover faster and breastfeed more easily. They want to connect intimately to the birth experience, which they believe will allow them to bond with their baby in an enhanced way. They believe a baby born without medical intervention will be calmer and more relaxed. The rediscovered enthusiasm for home births has accelerated in recent years as some women worry that they won't be able to achieve a peaceful birth experience on a maternity ward. With strangers running in and out of the rooms, nurses asking one another about other patients, and a multitude of intrusive machines, the ability to create an intimate, personalized environment in a hospital setting is difficult.

Other moms believe that pregnancy and labor need to be monitored carefully. They recognize that things can go wrong despite the best-laid plans and don't want to take any chances. They admit that labor is too painful to go through it without an epidural and appreciate being able to rest and save their strength for taking care of their newborn. They feel reassured that an operating room is right around the corner. They find comfort in knowing that a pediatrician is readily available if their baby needs any assistance. They know they will have the energy to focus on their baby after the less stressful experience of a medicated birth. They recognize that what feels good may not always be what is safest.

The conflict between natural and interventional birth extends to doctors and midwives as well, who philosophically look at childbirth differently. A doctor is trained to view pregnancy as a medical event and to look for the smallest deviations from the norm that could signal something is wrong. Doctors try to eliminate or at least minimize risks by performing tests, monitoring the mother regularly, and utilizing all of the latest technology.

A midwife views birth as a normal process that women's bodies are designed to undertake without difficulty. She believes that patience will allow nature to take its course. Although these philosophies are different, the goal is the same: to manage the unpredictability of birth.

Deciding What Is Right for You

the doctor's diary

If I could give you only one piece of advice, it would be to do what makes you happy. In a world where there is so much pressure to be a specific type of mother, it would be nice to go through pregnancy and childbirth the way you want. Not the way your friend did it, or the way the judgmental woman in line with you at Starbucks would.

As with most decisions in medicine, each of your choices in childbirth will have its own risks and benefits. I believe that natural childbirth can be an amazing, beautiful experience. However, it is not for everyone. Some women have no interest in it whatsoever, get every intervention possible, and still have a wonderful experience.

I believe that many women don't pursue a natural birth because we—the obstetrical community—have set them up to fail at it. Many things we do—some of which have no proven benefit—make it nearly impossible to achieve a natural delivery. We don't give women the tools they need to be successful, which only leads to disappointment—the last thing you need as a new mom. Follow your instincts, ask lots of questions, and stand up for what is important to you.

How do you decide which type of birth is right for you? Some women have a clear vision even before they get pregnant. Others aren't so sure. Natural sounds great but they fear that the pain will be more than they can handle. Some women know they want an epidural as soon as they get to the hospital. Still others plan to do whatever their doctor suggests in the moment.

When considering your options, you must think realistically about your health, your personal risk factors, and your fitness. Do you have a low-risk pregnancy, or do you have a medical condition that cannot be ignored? Has your blood pressure been slowly climbing upward from week to week? Has your baby suddenly done a somersault and is now breech with only a month left in the pregnancy? Are you significantly overweight? When you've spent months preparing for a certain type of birth and you have your heart set on a particular outcome, it's tempting to continue in that direction although it may not be safe.

the doctor's diary

I know from personal experience that not all births go as planned. When I was pregnant with my first baby at age thirty-four, I planned to continue my obstetrical practice until the moment I had to run upstairs to the hospital, deliver my son, and get right into the swing of motherhood without losing a beat. I was sure I'd be the model of natural birth; I was healthy, fit, and prepared. So, I was completely caught off guard when I developed severe preeclampsia (high blood pressure) at twenty-nine weeks. Because I had no symptoms and felt completely normal, I insisted that the blood pressure cuff must be broken as I saw the numbers climb over 200/110 (normal blood pressure is 120/80). Even with my pressure sky-high, I tried to negotiate a plan with my doctor so I could go home and wait for labor to ensue at the normal time. Instead, I found myself on bed rest in the hospital for two weeks, followed by an induction, an epidural, and a magnesium-induced haze from the medication I was given to prevent seizures. My son was born at thirty-one weeks, weighing 3 pounds 12 ounces, and was whisked off to the neonatal intensive care unit (NICU) without my even being able to touch him. It was exactly the opposite of the experience I had planned.

The truth is, some things just happen in the course of pregnancy that change your level of risk, and there's nothing you can do to prevent it. In my own case, I finally accepted my high-risk status. Thankfully, despite a small bleed in his brain, my son overcame the challenges of prematurity and is a healthy, thriving teenager.

When I look back on the delivery of my son, I feel both disappointed and grateful. I had hoped to hold him right after he was born, to breast-feed, to get to know him in the delivery room. But instead, I could only touch him through the holes in the Plexiglas incubator for weeks. We tell women that they should hope for a healthy mom and a healthy baby at the end—that should be enough. Isn't that the definition of a successful childbirth experience? I had that, yet it wasn't enough to eliminate the disappointment that I had a high-risk pregnancy and couldn't have the birth I wanted. At the same time, I feel grateful that I had access to prenatal care that allowed me to find out about my condition before I was too sick. I was also thankful that my son could live in a state-of-the-art NICU where the incubator and high-tech medical care allowed him to grow.

Whereas some risk factors develop during pregnancy, others appear only once you are in the delivery room in labor. Everything has been going along smoothly, until you find out that your baby is stuck in one position and can't rotate through the birth canal. Or that every time you have a contraction, the baby's heart rate dips because it has inadvertently tied a knot in the umbilical cord. There is no way to predict how a pregnancy will conclude. For this reason, doctors categorize pregnancies as low risk or high risk—there's no such thing as a "no-risk" pregnancy.

Women with low-risk pregnancies have many options for childbirth. If you and your doctor or midwife have determined that you are truly low risk, you can choose a noninterventional birth. You should fully commit to preparing for this during pregnancy. It means intensive education, reading, classes, and reflection. You can't just arrive in the delivery room and say, "I don't want this, I don't want that," without preparing yourself for how you will deal with the realities of labor. Most women who plan for an unmedicated birth attend childbirth classes for at least a few months. They may hire a doula to provide them with continuous emotional support during labor. They eat well and they stay fit. They consider what helps them to relax and prepare accordingly.

Planning for the birthing style you want is where your relationship with your doctor or midwife really counts. Your provider can help you determine what is safest for your individual situation. Hopefully, you will work with someone whom you trust, someone who will listen to your concerns and not dismiss what is important to you. When a mother feels supported, rather than managed, she will have an easier birth. Your labor may take an unexpected turn but your doctor can help you stay on the track you have chosen.

Ultimately, childbirth can be anything: overwhelming, guilt-ridden, beautiful, agonizing, calm, enlightening. I can think of no other life experience that brings out such diametrically opposite emotions—sometimes at the same time. As you think about what you want your birth to be like, you may find yourself overcome with fear or doubt. Remember that every woman has felt the same way at some point in her pregnancy. Odds are you're a lot more capable than you give yourself credit for. Frame your own narrative by listening to the positive stories. Focus on bringing your baby into the world with your loving family cheering you on. And support other women in their choices, whether or not they mirror yours. Stay clear-eyed, with an open mind and an open heart: you're on your way to becoming a mother.

SCIENCE, EMOTION, AND TRADITION

—and How They Influence Your Ob-Gyn

HEALTHY MOM, HEALTHY BABY. IT SEEMS LIKE A STRAIGHT-forward goal. While your provider has your best interests and those of your baby at heart, she must contend with a number of external factors that influence your care during pregnancy and delivery. Basic scientific knowledge about how the body works and how to diagnose and treat complications is a starting point. But there are also intangibles that affect her medical recommendations, ranging from where she completed her residency to whether she has ever been named in a malpractice lawsuit. Even the structure of her private practice—whether she has a partner who can lend a hand when she is attending a delivery—can influence her advice.

Medical decisions are not simply a matter of what is safest or wisest, or what has been proven in a medical study. We doctors also take into account how our patient and her family are going to feel

11

about our approach, how other health-care workers on the team will see things, what our colleagues would do, what is convenient, and unfortunately, what could happen in a lawsuit if something goes wrong. Medical decision-making is a complicated intertwining of science, emotions, and traditions. These considerations often prevent optimal care. However, if you are aware of these "nonmedical" factors, you can collaborate with your doctor to resolve problems in a way that is a win-win for everyone.

The Powers That Be

The American College of Obstetricians and Gynecologists (ACOG) sets the standards for ob-gyns in practice and has fifty-eight thousand members. The organization keeps physicians up to date on the latest medical research and provides evidence-based recommendations on how to treat patients. It sponsors clinical and scientific meetings where physicians and researchers can present their latest data to colleagues. It publishes *Committee Opinions* on a wide range of topics, such as "Cell-free DNA Screening" to "Marijuana Use in Pregnancy," so doctors can be kept apprised of the latest research in the field. Beyond disseminating research data, the organization releases *Practice Bulletins*, which explain the basis and evidence for medical recommendations. These publications cover such topics as "Management of Gestational Diabetes," "Prevention of Preterm Birth," and "The Use of Psychiatric Drugs During Pregnancy."

Because the guidelines set forth by ACOG rely on research, clinical trials, and reporting from members, most doctors believe they represent the best practices for treating their patients. If a doctor ignores ACOG's recommendations, he may not only be providing you with substandard care, but he is also opening himself up to criticism from his peers and malpractice lawsuits.

On numerous occasions, patients have asked me to deviate from the standard of care set forth by ACOG. I want my patients to have the birth they desire, to have a healthy baby, and to look back on the experience in a positive way. If I "take a risk" with them, I find myself in a dilemma between what would make my patient happy and what the medical community says is acceptable.

For example, the current standard is to perform a cesarean if a woman has been pushing for more than three hours and has been unable to deliver the baby. She may insist that she wants to avoid a cesarean, and asks me whether she can continue to push longer. If I say no, she will never know whether she could have done it, will feel disappointed, and probably have a negative view of me, believing that I did not support her. If I say yes and she continues to push to delivery, but her baby has a complication, such as a shoulder dystocia, I am responsible for that decision.

Other situations in which a patient has asked me to do something outside of standard practices include:

- Declining a diabetes screening test
- Wanting a vaginal birth after cesarean (VBAC) following two previous cesareans
- Going more than two weeks past the due date without induction of labor
- Not wanting IV antibiotics for Group B strep infection
- Wanting to deliver a breech baby vaginally
- Wanting to continue to labor when the baby's heart rate shows signs of distress

As much as I may want to be the "good guy," I feel pressured to stay within the ACOG guidelines even if I personally believe that a certain path may be perfectly safe.

See One, Do One, Teach One

How an ob-gyn is trained during residency greatly influences how he practices throughout his career. Most training takes place in teaching hospitals that are affiliated with universities, but some are in smaller community hospitals. Teaching hospitals expose future ob-gyns to high-risk pregnancies, rare diseases, and numerous complications of labor, which lead many new doctors to view pregnancy as a disease to be assessed, tested, and resolved. Instruction is done by professors who are physicians with administrative duties, patient responsibilities, and research projects. In addition, much of the training is done by the older residents. The motto is: "See one, do one, teach one." That means that on the first day of residency, a new doctor will "catch" her first baby. By the end of the same day, she may be showing another new doctor how to do the same. In this way, skills and habits—both good and bad—are passed from one group of residents to the next.

A resident seeks to develop a diverse wealth of knowledge as well as advanced surgical skills. As a result, the focus moves away from the patient's experience of her birth. Under these circumstances, it is rare to observe a birth that doesn't have some sort of intervention. In fact, because residents need to fulfill training requirements, they are eager to practice their skills such as using forceps and vacuum, or performing cesareans.

Residents usually work in shifts, often lasting twenty-four to thirty hours at a time. Since 2003, residents are restricted to working eighty hours per week. They work on labor and delivery for a month or two, and then move on to other aspects of their training, such as gynecology or infertility, returning to deliver babies again a few months later. A resident obstetrician, on average, will attend 273 vaginal deliveries and 232 C-sections during the four-year training program.

Maintaining a continuity of care is an ongoing struggle for these doctors-in-training. They rarely know a patient from the beginning of her pregnancy to her delivery. A resident often meets his patient for the first time on the labor and delivery unit without having established a relationship with her or her family. He manages her labor during his 24-hour shift. Then a new physician will come on. As a result, continuity of care—for the doctor and the patient—is lacking. The first doctor is not around to see what happened during the delivery and the second doctor didn't participate in the decision-making early on.

During residency, practice patterns are established. New doctors are molded by their professors and classmates on everything from which type of suture to use to sew up a uterus to how long to wait to induce labor. If a resident observes others using episiotomies on a regular basis, he is more likely to do so as well. If he is taught to perform a cesarean when there is a certain pattern of fetal distress, he will continue that practice for years to come. The subtleties and nuances of the art of obstetrics are established during this significant time.

On Call

Sixty-five percent of ob-gyns enter private practice after residency. In private practice, the doctor you see during the pregnancy is the same person who attends your delivery. The benefit of this model is the strength of the doctor-patient relationship. Seeing only one provider throughout the nine months and having that doctor manage your labor assures that he understands your medical condition as well as your wishes and desires for the birth. For the doctor, it is also the ultimate payoff, and one of the best parts of practicing obstetrics. Getting to know a family for many months and then being present at the most exciting day of their journey is incredibly rewarding.

Doctors have the option of working in a solo practice or joining a group. Most groups work out a schedule of being "on call" so that doctors cover for one another at night and on the weekends. During office hours, if one doctor needs to leave for a delivery, another may step in to see the patients waiting.

In reality, the private practice model is a difficult lifestyle to sustain. If a doctor is going to be available to deliver each of his patients, he also needs to find a way to manage the unpredictable, exhausting, and unique schedule that is inherent to this field. Your doctor is "on call" every night or every few nights for years or decades on end.

Typically, he receives multiple phone calls in the middle of the night and may need to go to the hospital for a birth. Sleepless nights are followed by a full schedule of patients in the office the next day.

Ob-gyns struggle to balance the needs of a woman in labor with those of the patients in the office who have appointments. As a result, an ob-gyn cannot be at the bedside during all of labor. Instead he is updated regularly on the patient's condition by the nurse on the phone, who may even push with her patient nearly to the point that the baby is ready to deliver. Then the nurse will instruct the mother to stop pushing, wait, and breathe until the doctor arrives.

Even more challenging for obstetricians is making personal commitments, such as taking their own children to school, having dinner with family and friends, or attending a soccer game. Without a doubt, an ob-gyn will miss many important events due to the demands of this specialty. This sacrifice is generally balanced by the joy and satisfaction the doctor receives from it. However, OBs in busy practices "burn out" at a younger age than other medical specialties. The average age for an ob-gyn to stop delivering babies (and practice only gynecology) is forty-nine.

The demanding schedule of private practice leads doctors to recommend interventions that can speed up the delivery, such as breaking the water bag or coaching a patient on how to push instead of allowing her to do it instinctively. Although doctors may not want to admit it, many cesareans have been performed because the doctor had another patient in labor, he needed to get back to the office, or he simply wanted to go to sleep.

Protocols, Policies, and Rules

Hospitals set protocols for labor and delivery that doctors and staff must follow. These rules are meant to ensure the safety and best outcomes for the patients. Each labor and delivery unit has hundreds of policies—how often vital signs are recorded, how to dispose of unused medication, how a fetus should be monitored during labor, and how many visitors can be in the operating room for a cesarean. A committee of doctors, nurses, and hospital employees revise the protocols every few years as medical standards change.

Some common protocols make achieving natural childbirth more difficult. For example, the Joint Commission on Accreditation of Healthcare Organizations (JCAHO) has developed formal standards for the care, assessment, and management of pain for hospitalized patients. While pain is a known and necessary component of labor, it is not acceptable for patients in other areas of the hospital. Yet, the protocols apply to all patients equally. These guidelines say that:

- All individuals have the right to pain management.
- Nurses must assess the existence, nature, and intensity of pain in all patients.
- Hospitals must establish policies for ordering effective medication.
- Nurses and doctors must educate patients about pain medicine options.

A woman wanting an unmedicated birth may prefer not to be asked about her pain or offered pain medications because frequently turning her attention to the concept of "pain" may cause her to lose focus and abandon her natural relaxation techniques. In the hospital setting, ignoring this protocol is not an option.

Additional protocols and rules on labor and delivery may include the following:

- You can't eat or drink during labor.
- You must have an IV.
- Your partner can't be in the room while you get an epidural.
- You must stay in bed after your water has broken.
- Your other children aren't allowed in the delivery room.
- If a certain number of hours have passed after water has broken, labor must be induced.

- Your family can't take pictures or video.
- Your baby's heart rate must be monitored continuously.
- Your baby will be taken for an assessment and a bath immediately after birth.

While hospital protocols define some of the details of your experience, they do not dictate whether your doctor should or shouldn't perform a cesarean. This decision is ultimately made by the doctor alone, not the hospital nor its administration, and is based on his assessment of you. In rare cases, hospital staff, such as a nurse or another physician, may intervene on behalf of a patient if they think that a colleague is doing something unsafe.

Staying on the Right Side of the Law

Threats of a malpractice lawsuit impact how your doctor manages your pregnancy, labor, and delivery. By practicing conservatively, she hopes not only to provide excellent care but to avoid an outcome that could result in a malpractice case. However, the fear of litigation does not necessarily help doctors deliver healthier babies. Instead, it leads to defensive medicine that disrupts the bond between patient and physician.

Lawsuits in medicine are common, with sixteen thousand new malpractice cases filed every year. Sixty-one percent of all doctors, and 78 percent of ob-gyns, will be sued at least once. In fact, ob-gyns are sued, on average, 2.64 times during their career. Each malpractice claim takes about five years to reach a conclusion. While 40 percent of the cases are eventually dropped, 40 percent are settled before trial and 20 percent go to court. The average financial award to the plaintiff is $500,000.

All physicians who work in a hospital must carry malpractice insurance. Malpractice insurance premiums vary tremendously from state to state and are based on each state's laws regarding malpractice award limits. An ob-gyn in Minnesota will pay $17,000 per year,

MOST COMMON REASONS FOR
MALPRACTICE LAWSUITS IN OBSTETRICS

A doctor's goal for your pregnancy and childbirth is for you to have a healthy baby. Unfortunately, sometimes things go wrong and a child is injured, born with an undiagnosed illness, or does not survive. The most common malpractice claims are due to:

- Cerebral palsy: This permanent neuro-muscular disorder causes difficulties in walking, speaking, and swallowing due to an abnormality in the part of the brain controlling movement. It usually develops during pregnancy but can also be due to an injury during childbirth.
- Failure to diagnose a condition such as a birth defect
- Shoulder dystocia and brachial plexus injury: After the baby's head delivers, the shoulders become stuck. While dislodging the shoulder, the baby's neck stretches, which can permanently damage the nerves to the arm and hand.
- Stillbirth: A baby who dies during pregnancy or childbirth
- Complication of a VBAC or operative delivery

whereas one in Florida will pay over $200,000. In the United States, $7 billion per year is spent on malpractice insurance premiums. In addition, the cost of the practice of defensive medicine and the changes in physician behavior in response to the threat of lawsuits is estimated at $100 billion per year.

One reason for the high cesarean rate in the United States is the fear of malpractice. Over 70 percent of all claims—such as those for cerebral palsy, shoulder dystocia, stillbirth, and complications of a VBAC—are related to a doctor's failure to perform a cesarean. In this legal environment, many doctors believe that if there is the slightest concern about a baby's health, there is no justification for *not* doing a C-section. Until patients stop suing doctors for failing to perform cesareans, doctors will continue to do them. Cesarean rates vary from state to state, but they are highest in states with the most malpractice lawsuits and highest insurance premiums, such as Florida and New

York. For every increase in a doctor's malpractice insurance premium by $10,000, the C-section rate increases by 1.6 percent.

An ACOG survey on professional liability from 2012 surveyed nine thousand ob-gyns and found that 51 percent admitted they changed the way they practice to avoid lawsuits by only taking care of low-risk patients. Some acknowledged that they performed more C-sections. Others stopped offering VBACs.

The Business of Birth

About 4 million babies are born each year in the United States, making pregnancy and childbirth an industry in itself. In 2012, the cost of prenatal care with a vaginal birth averaged $18,329; with a cesarean section, $27,866. Well over $50 billion per year is spent on maternity and newborn care, the highest in the world. The United States has more tests, older mothers, more cesareans and inductions, more uninsured patients, and higher malpractice premiums. Many US patients, thinking that they will get better care, insist on seeing an obstetrician at every prenatal visit and want a doctor to deliver their baby as well. In other countries, midwives handle low-risk pregnancies, which keeps costs down.

BIRTH BY THE NUMBERS

As of this writing, this is the average hospital cost for a vaginal birth—*not including prenatal care*—in a sampling of developed countries:

United States	$9,775
Australia	$6,800
Switzerland	$4,039
France	$3,541
Netherlands	$2,669
United Kingdom	$2,641
Spain	$2,200
Argentina	$1,200

Your doctor is paid a "global fee" for obstetrical care. This payment covers all of your prenatal care, delivery, and postpartum visits, and is the same amount whether you see the doctor five times or fifteen times during the pregnancy. With most HMO insurance and Medicaid, the global fee for a vaginal birth is the same as for a cesarean. If you have preferred provider option (PPO) insurance, your doctor may receive slightly higher compensation (an extra $200) for a cesarean. Global fees vary by location. They may be as low as $900 for Medicaid and up to $3,500 for some PPO plans.

the doctor's diary

Patients have told me that they assume doctors and hospitals want to perform cesareans to make more money. I can assure you it's not about the money. While a cesarean may provide a little more compensation with some insurance plans, it's not enough to be an incentive. However, delivering the baby quickly does allow the doctor to move on to the next delivery or patient in the office, which may indirectly influence him financially. Similarly, while a hospital receives a higher payment for a cesarean, the extra supplies, monitors, and nursing staff needed to care for the patient after surgery erase any significant profit.

Medical decision-making reflects sound principles of science, safety, and ethical practice. An ob-gyn strives to give his patients the best possible care within the boundaries of his profession. However, many factors shape your doctor's perspective and his ability to follow a plan that meets your expectations. Some of the influences on your doctor's practice are subconscious, such as the way he was trained. Others are concrete rules established by hospitals. All of these color your experience of birth in different ways, some of which are contrary to what you may have envisioned. Talk with your doctor about your goals and whether there may be any policies or circumstances that inhibit their being realized. By understanding how your doctor makes decisions, and the protocols and practices he must follow, you can work together to reach agreements on how to make your pregnancy and birth as safe as it can be.

NATURAL CHOICES

—about Eating, Exercise, Environment, and More

FINDING OUT YOU ARE EXPECTING BRINGS JOY AND EXCITEMENT about a new chapter in your life. But the journey from that positive pregnancy test to a baby in your arms can be complicated. It's normal to have concerns and fears about the pregnancy, the health of the baby, and giving birth. You may be afraid of having a miscarriage, of delivering early, or that something you've done will hurt your baby.

Information about pregnancy and childbirth can be found everywhere—in books, on mommy blogs and websites, and in social media. For every website saying that something is safe, there's another one saying the same thing is dangerous. One pregnancy book says you should eat lots of fish for the omega-3 fatty acids; another says fish contains mercury that will poison your baby and lead to birth defects. Don't have children too young; don't have children too old. The contradictions are endless, and for a woman who wants to do everything she can to ensure the health of her baby, overwhelming.

Scientific discoveries that help us understand pregnancy also cause distress in new moms by revealing numerous things that can go wrong. You can now be screened for hundreds of genetic mutations. Ultrasounds identify small irregularities in the fetus that may be associated with serious problems, but also may be completely normal. Electronic fetal monitoring shows fluctuations in a baby's heartbeat that may or may not have any significance. These days, it seems that there is something to be concerned about in nearly every pregnancy.

the doctor's diary

How did we become so afraid in pregnancy? I know each mom is merely trying her best to navigate the world of conflicting advice. She is making decisions for two, and takes her role seriously. No electric blankets or microwaves. No sushi or hot dogs. No high heels or nail polish. While I find some of these recommendations amusing at best, I know that my patients want to do what is right and feel immensely confused when confronted with contradictory information about what is safe—and what is not. For those who want the short version of the scientifically proven things you can do to benefit your baby, here's my top 10 list:

- Manage your stress.
- Maintain a normal weight before conceiving.
- Buy organic or wash your produce meticulously.
- Cook meats thoroughly.
- Eat lots of fish.
- Exercise vigorously and regularly.
- Minimize your alcohol intake.
- Don't smoke.
- Wash your hands frequently if you have children or are exposed to illnesses.
- Discuss any medications with your doctor.

Should You Stress About Stress?

Many moms-to-be are concerned about the effect that stress may have on their developing baby. Being pregnant doesn't shield you from the pressures and challenges of everyday life, such as a death in the family, marital problems, difficulties on the job, or financial strains. In fact, pregnancy itself can be the cause of tension. You worry whether the baby is healthy. You consider how you will manage a work schedule while taking care of a newborn. As it turns out, taking steps to reduce stress is just as important as stopping smoking and eating well.

For generations, pregnant women were treated as fragile. In some cultures, being pregnant meant you were not allowed to lift heavy things, exercise, or work. People believed that stress could cause a miscarriage, hurt the baby, or cause a woman to go into labor early. However, in the 1960s, experts acknowledged that the scientific evidence didn't support this theory, and dismissed as folklore the proviso that pregnant women should "take it easy." Pregnant women found themselves working full-time, being on their feet all day, and staying active until the moment that labor started. More recently, however, the philosophy on stress during pregnancy has changed yet again in light of the revelations provided by a new field of science called epigenetics.

EPIGENETICS

Since the discovery of DNA in the 1950s, scientists have known that traits such as eye color, height, and propensity for developing certain diseases are determined by the specific genes we inherit from our parents. However, in the last two decades, further research has shown that our genes are not set in stone but can be altered by external and environmental factors during pregnancy. These factors modify the DNA without changing its sequence, such that cells "read" the DNA differently. Scientists termed the way diet, toxins, and other forces—including stress—alter our DNA *epigenetics*. Epigenetics is one way our body adapts to ensure survival. For example, if a woman is pregnant during a stressful time, it may benefit her child to be extra-sensitive to stress hormones so that he can also flourish in that environment, and the baby develops accordingly.

continues–

—continued

Epigenetics is particularly significant for a developing fetus,
suggesting that disease prevention actually begins in the womb.
Many of the studies on epigenetics are conducted in animal
models so, at this time, it is unclear whether these findings also
apply to humans. While there is not a definitive cause and effect,
there does appear to be an association between what a woman
does during pregnancy and who her child grows up to be.

Stress and Your Body

When you are stressed, your body secretes hormones, such as cortisol and catecholamines (adrenaline) that trigger the "fight or flight"
response. Your heart rate increases, blood flows to your muscles,
and you have a boost of energy. This reaction is meant to be tem-
porary. When these hormones remain elevated because the stress is
still present, they can have negative consequences, such as raising
blood sugar levels, decreasing the amount of oxygen being delivered
to tissues, and suppressing the immune system. Besides its direct
effects on the body, stress also leads to other unhealthy habits, such
as smoking, drinking alcohol, or not eating and sleeping well.

During pregnancy, these hormones decrease the blood supply to
the uterus and fetus. This effect is seen when a pregnant woman is
physically as well as emotionally stressed. In addition, the placenta
makes its own unique hormone in response to stress, called corti-
cotropin-releasing hormone (CRH). High levels of CRH are linked
to premature deliveries.

How Much Stress Is Too Much?

Normal everyday stressors do not impact a pregnancy, but long-
term burdens may. These include starvation, having another child
with a chronic illness, living in crowded conditions, unemployment,

and having poor coping skills. A specific life-changing event, such as the death of a partner or child, or a diagnosis of cancer or other serious illness, can also have a significant effect. A pregnancy is less vulnerable to stress during its later stages, whereas those during the first trimester have the greatest impact. For example, after the 6.7 magnitude Northridge earthquake in 1994, more babies were born prematurely to mothers who were in the first trimester when the event occurred.[1]

In addition to life events, a woman's overall anxiety levels, ability to relax, and personality traits, such as neuroticism, may affect who her child grows up to be. A woman who is generally nervous, has poor coping skills, or is depressed may be at the highest risk for having an anxious child.[2]

Effect of Stress on Pregnancy

- Low birth weight: Chronic stress is associated with low birth weight babies.
- Preterm labor: The risk of preterm birth is doubled in cases of severe stress.
- Birth defects: Stressful life events increase the risk of cleft lip and congenital heart disease.
- Future health of child: Maternal stress may affect a child's overall health and susceptibility to disease later in life. It has also been linked to depression, irritability, problems with attention, and lower IQ.

Learning to Relax

Just because you have a stressful life doesn't mean you will have a complication in your pregnancy or a child with behavioral problems. If you find ways to cope with your stress and diffuse it effectively, you can have a perfectly healthy pregnancy and baby.

─────────────── **RESEARCH SPOTLIGHT** ───────────────

Fascinating research on stress and health conducted by Sonja Entringer was published in an article in *Current Opinion in Endocrinology, Diabetes and Obesity* in December 2010.[3] Inside all our cells, DNA is arranged in bundles called chromosomes. At the ends of the chromosomes are areas called telomeres, which are like the plastic tips on the end of a shoelace. Telomeres protect our genes and help cells divide properly. As a cell divides, the telomeres shorten to a critical point, and the cell dies. Short telomeres are associated with premature aging, heart disease, diabetes, and cancer. People with extended telomeres live for an average of five years longer than do those with short telomeres.

Telomere length is influenced by the cumulative stress during a lifetime. In addition, maternal stress may "program" the telomere system of the developing fetus. Women who are stressed during pregnancy give birth to babies with shorter telomeres, affecting their future health.

Stress reduction should be an integral part of prenatal care. Doctors are reluctant to emphasize the link between stress and poor pregnancy outcomes because it is hard to determine exactly how much stress is too much. They worry that the discussion itself may lead women to experience anxiety about hurting their babies. But asking about stress may have as much significance as measuring blood pressure or listening to the baby's heart rate in assuring a good outcome for both the woman and her fetus. Stress-reduction programs offering education, more frequent prenatal visits, and psychological support are shown to reduce the rate of preterm births by 19 percent.[4]

For pregnant women, some simple strategies to cope with or reduce stress, such as yoga, exercise, support groups, and prenatal education, may help. The sources of stress must be carefully identified and actions taken to cope with or reduce it. If the workplace is a source of unmanageable stress, if economically feasible, it may be necessary to take a leave of absence until the baby is born.

Stress Relief During Pregnancy

• Talk about it with your partner, doctor, friends.
• Modify your work schedule.
• Exercise and sleep more.
• Educate yourself about what to expect during pregnancy and childbirth. Take birthing classes.
• Be prepared for the reality that some aspects of pregnancy are out of your control. If you have nausea, bleeding, or preterm labor, you may need to modify your work schedule.
• Learn relaxation techniques, such as meditation, and give yourself permission to take the time to use them.
• See a therapist.

Depression During Pregnancy

It is normal to feel emotional during pregnancy. Your body is flooded with hormones and your life is about to change dramatically. Your emotions can range from thrilled to overwhelmed and anxious. However, when the symptoms of sadness and feeling withdrawn persist and dominate your life, you may be clinically depressed. One in five women are depressed during their pregnancy. More than half of these will also develop postpartum depression.

If you have any of these symptoms for more than two weeks, you should contact a mental health professional:

• Difficulty sleeping
• Loss of energy
• Inability to concentrate
• Loss of appetite
• Decreased interest in activities
• Feeling guilty
• Thoughts of suicide

Five Things You Need to Know About Depression

1. Depression in pregnancy should always be treated with medication, therapy, or both.

2. Depression has been linked to preterm births and poor fetal growth, similar to the effects of stress. Untreated depression can also affect the psychological development of your baby, resulting in irritability as an infant and depression and behavioral issues during childhood and the teen years.

3. If you are being treated for depression prior to pregnancy, you should talk with your doctor about your medications. Most antidepressants are safe, but a few—Prozac and Paxil—have been linked to certain birth defects. You should consider tapering off those medications altogether and switching to a different antidepressant, such as Zoloft, Lexapro, or Celexa.[5]

4. You should not abruptly stop any antidepressants, because you may relapse. If your symptoms are mild, your doctor can taper your medication over one to three months and treat you with therapy alone. But if your depression is significant, you should stay on medication throughout the pregnancy.

5. Treatment for depression in pregnancy is successful in 90 percent of women. The earlier that treatment is started, the quicker the recovery.

Optimize Your Health

Along with attending to your emotional well-being, maintaining a nutritious diet, along with exercise, is a great way to be sure that you and your growing baby get what you need. Ideally, you should improve your eating habits prior to becoming pregnant, but if you are already pregnant, there is a lot you can do to stay healthy.

Weighing In: Your Starting Point

Of course, every mom strives to be her best when she's planning to become pregnant. She wants to eat well, be fit and healthy, and be at an ideal weight. Believe it or not, even more important than how much weight you gain during pregnancy is whether you are overweight or obese when you start. Obesity automatically makes your pregnancy "high risk" because of the propensity for developing complications. The chance you will need a cesarean is nearly 50 percent.

- Risks for mothers:
    Miscarriage
    Gestational diabetes
    Preeclampsia,
    Having a large baby
- Risk to babies:
    Prematurity
    Stillbirth
    Birth defects such as neural tube defects
    Childhood obesity
- Risks during labor:
    Difficult monitoring the baby's heart rate
    Difficult epidural placement
    Shoulder dystocia
    Need for cesarean
- The cesarean rate increases with BMI:

BMI	Cesarean rate
Less than 30	21%
30–35	34%
Greater than 35	47%

- Risks with cesarean:
    Increased blood loss
    Infection
    Blood clots
    Injury to surrounding organs

Nauseous One Minute, Ravenous the Next

There is no aspect of pregnancy advice more riddled with myths than that relating to what you should and shouldn't eat. The mommy police are hard at work, chastising other women in sushi bars and coffee shops. Googling "pregnancy diet" leads to hundreds of websites with recommendations that contradict one another: Avoid sushi at all costs. Don't drink coffee or carbonated drinks. Don't eat anything spicy. The warnings are everywhere and are rarely based on any sort of science. The truth is that the best diet for a pregnant woman reflects the basic principles of healthy eating that we all know. It involves eating lots of fruits and vegetables, lean proteins, and whole grains, and avoiding processed foods, fried foods, and excessive sugar.

Advice about how many calories you should be consuming is also fraught with misconceptions. Thankfully, the idea of "eating for two" has finally gone by the wayside. Much to the chagrin of moms who would like to use pregnancy as an excuse to overindulge, that suggestion never made sense because you obviously aren't eating for another adult. However, since almost half of all pregnant women gain more weight than is recommended, the messages they are receiving about calorie intake are either inaccurate or ineffective. Total calorie intake should increase by 200 to 300 calories per day, but only during the last twelve weeks of pregnancy. Your basal metabolic rate (BMR)—how many calories your body burns at rest—stays the same during the first half of pregnancy. The BMR doesn't significantly increase until thirty-two weeks. In addition, during the first and second trimesters, your body's metabolism changes so that you absorb more calories and nutrients from the same amount of food. It is only when the baby is growing larger in the third trimester that you need any extra calories.

While you may alternate between feeling nauseous and ravenous, especially at the beginning of pregnancy, this is not a signal that you need to eat more. Instead, a complex interaction of hormones, including progesterone, insulin, leptin, and ghrelin, cause you to feel constantly hungry. Answering your cravings with proteins and low-fat foods will make you feel satisfied and stave off excessive weight gain.

At each prenatal visit, your provider will measure your weight. He does this, in most cases, not because he's concerned that you aren't gaining enough but that you are gaining too much. You can ignore the pregnancy books and websites that outline specific "pounds per week" goals. You don't need to gain a certain amount of weight per trimester. You should eat to satiety when you are hungry without feeling stuffed. The changes in your body's metabolism will do the rest.

Your *maximum* weight gain depends on your starting point. If you are:

Normal weight: Your maximum weight gain should be 30 pounds.
Underweight: Your maximum weight gain should be 35 pounds.
Overweight: Your maximum weight gain should be 20 pounds.
Obese: Your maximum weight gain should be 15 pounds.

Exceeding these limits puts you at risk for having a large baby, needing a cesarean, developing gestational diabetes, and struggling to lose the weight after delivery.

Eating "Clean" and Natural

Women who are pregnant should focus on eating unprocessed whole foods, including grains, fruits, vegetables, meat, and dairy. Families should try to do their own cooking during pregnancy to control what they are eating and to know the source of their food. Organic foods are an excellent choice because they do not contain pesticides, growth hormones, antibiotics, or fertilizers. Of course, eating organic can be expensive. Organic foods cost 50 to 100 percent more than the nonorganic version. If you can't afford to buy organic, you should peel your fruits and vegetables or wash them for at least thirty seconds before eating. Farmers' markets may have less costly options for organically grown foods than a natural foods or grocery store. Be sure to ask vendors whether the produce was grown organically, as their presence at a farmers' market only suggests freshness, not necessarily growing practices. In grocery stores, look on the label for an SKU starting with 9, to be sure the produce is organically grown. You can also check out https://www.ewg.org/foodnews/: every year, the Environmental Working Group posts the "dirty dozen"—the twelve types of produce you should avoid if grown conventionally—as well as the "clean fifteen"—the conventionally grown produce that's safe to eat.

GMOs (genetically modified organisms) were first introduced into our food supply in the 1990s, and now are found in 90 percent of the food we eat. A GMO is formed by taking the genes of one organism and forcing them into the genes of an unrelated organism. The most common GMOs insert genes into crops to make them resistant to herbicides, so farmers can kill weeds without harming the crops themselves. They also use GMOs to make crops produce their own pesticides. Nearly all the soy, canola, and corn grown in the United States contain GMOs.

The USDA considers GMOs as "generally recognized as safe" during pregnancy. A recent study in *Reproductive Toxicology*[6] showed that pesticides made by GMOs are found in the blood of 93 percent of pregnant women as well as 80 percent of umbilical cord blood.

The controversy about GMOs is divisive. The USDA and food producers attest to its safety while other scientists claim that the increases in cancers and autism may be linked to these changes in our food supply. Currently, no laws mandate that genetically modified foods are tested for safety, especially in pregnancy. While many of these products have been around for decades with no obvious negative repercussions, it may be prudent to avoid them when possible. Increasingly, manufacturers are willingly labeling those products that are GMO-free; in addition, a new federal law mandates that labeling using statements or QR codes must be done in the near future. Natural foods stores may be your best source for such products.

Foods to Avoid

Some foods can be dangerous to a developing fetus because they can carry infections or toxins. The most notable foods to avoid during pregnancy are those that could be contaminated with the bacteria *Listeria* or *Toxoplasma*, such as uncooked or undercooked meats. Avoid consuming:

- Raw meat
- Smoked seafood, unless it is cooked in a casserole or canned
- Pâté
- Deli meats (can be consumed if heated)
- Fish containing high levels of mercury (swordfish, tilefish, shark, and mackerel). Tuna should be limited to 6 ounces per week or 2 small cans of tuna per week.

  A note about mercury: The mercury in a woman's body is related to the amount of fish she has eaten over the last few years, not the last few months. While the FDA recommends avoiding some fish in pregnancy, it admits that stopping the consumption for nine months won't lower mercury levels significantly. Researchers from the National Institutes of Health suggest that the benefits of eating fish on child development outweigh the risk of mercury and, therefore, limiting fish consumption during pregnancy is detrimental. Just be sure to avoid fish with the highest mercury levels, such as shark, king mackerel, tilefish, and swordfish. A good resource for the latest data is https://www.nrdc.org/stories/smart-seafood-buying-guide.

- Unpasteurized cheeses (queso blanco, Brie, feta, blue-veined). Cheese produced in the United States is pasteurized and therefore safe. Imported cheese and cheese from a farmers' market may not be, so check the label for confirmation.

Classic "food poisoning" can be distinguished from listeriosis or toxoplasmosis by its symptoms. Food poisoning, caused by such viruses as norovirus or such bacteria as *E. coli* and *Salmonella*, causes diarrhea, vomiting, and abdominal pain that typically last for 24 hours. While it may cause dehydration, it is not harmful to the developing fetus. Listeriosis and toxoplasmosis cause fevers, swollen lymph nodes, headaches, and muscle aches and usually don't have the gastrointestinal symptoms seen with food poisoning.

Foods on the "Safe" List

Despite the advice you read in other pregnancy books and websites, these foods are perfectly safe during pregnancy if stored and prepared properly.

- Sushi (unless it is prepared from seafood that is high in mercury). Sushi-grade fish is flash frozen, which kills parasites, making sushi one of the least common sources of food-borne illness. However, you should not consume raw fish from the supermarket that is not designated as "sushi-grade." This fish is intended to be cooked and has not been flash frozen. Freezing supermarket fish in your own freezer is not adequate to kill the parasites.
- Hot dogs (unless they are uncooked)
- Eggs (unless raw). See page 37 regarding egg allergy.

- Prepared salads from the deli
- Shellfish, such as shrimp, lobster, and crab
- Raw oysters, mussels, clams
- Drinks containing caffeine. A moderate amount of caffeine—200 to 300 mg per day (1 or 2 cups of coffee per day)—is perfectly safe; see page 52.
- Herbal tea
- Foods that are related to allergies, such as nuts, milk, wheat, and eggs. Patients (and doctors) have been concerned that eating these foods during pregnancy leads to allergies in children. However, evidence does not support this theory. In fact, a 2013 study shows just the opposite—eating nuts during pregnancy (provided you are not allergic to them yourself)—reduces the risk of nut allergies in your child.[7]

Specific Diet Considerations and Pregnancy

Many women follow a specific diet either out of choice or out of necessity, such as due to an underlying allergy or sensitivity.

Gluten-free: The gluten-free diet, followed by those with celiac disease, wheat allergies, or gluten-intolerance, eliminates any foods containing gluten, a protein found in wheat, rye, barley, related grains, and possibly oats (via cross-contamination). Wheat flour, which is fortified with folic acid and iron, has served as a major source of these nutrients in the typical American diet. Therefore, women who eat gluten-free may have deficiencies in these nutrients. In addition, they may have low fiber intake. These deficits can easily be remedied by eating beans, fruits, nuts, vegetables, and fish. Gluten-free vitamin supplements can also be used.

Macrobiotic: The principles of macrobiotic eating reflect a belief that food and food quality affects our health and happiness. Proponents of a macrobiotic diet recommend eating regularly, chewing food completely, and staying active, as well as avoiding processed food and most animal products. The macrobiotic diet contains beans, vegetables, brown rice, miso soup, fish, and nuts. Food should be prepared in wood or glass. Those following this diet may lack vitamin B_{12}, calcium, iron, and vitamin D. These nutrients can be acquired by adding a supplement or making adjustments to the diet.

Vegan: The vegan diet consists of food derived from plants and does not contain any animal products or by-products (no meat, dairy, or eggs). It may be low in protein, DHA, calcium, and vitamins A, D, and B_{12}. In fact, 83 percent of vegans are deficient in vitamin B_{12}. Vegan pregnant women can consume extra protein through protein bars, nuts, lentils or other legumes, and soy milk or nut milks. Calcium can be found in broccoli, kale, and other cruciferous vegetables, and calcium-fortified nondairy milk. Vegans may also need to take a vitamin B_{12} supplement, since this vitamin is found only in animal products.

Vegetarian: The vegetarian diet eliminates meats but may include eggs and/or dairy products. This diet may also be deficient in DHA and vitamins A, D, and B_{12}. Vegetarians can supplement DHA by eating flaxseeds, dark green vegetables, and yogurt.

Paleo: A paleo diet seeks to mimic the foods eaten by early humans, including meats, fish, fruits, and vegetables. It avoids dairy, processed foods, and grains. Most vitamins and minerals are easily attained through this diet, so there is no need for supplements during pregnancy.

Supplements

There isn't a pregnancy website, book, or doctor that doesn't tell you to take your prenatal vitamins. It seems to be the one topic that everyone can agree on. However, if you are eating a well-balanced diet of nutrient-rich foods, you will receive all the vitamins and minerals that you need through these daily meals. In fact, vitamins and minerals that are found in food are better absorbed than those in supplements, so making changes to your diet is the best place to start to ensure you are getting everything you need for your baby. There is no medical evidence that taking a prenatal vitamin improves the outcome of your pregnancy.

If you want to take a prenatal supplement, how do you know which products are best? Drugstores stock shelf after shelf with vitamins and supplements. There are so many options for prenatal vitamins that a woman planning her pregnancy may not know where to begin. You can find vitamins that are tiny or chewable, liquid or chocolate-flavored. Some are kosher and others help with nausea. Do you need that extra DHA? What about a stool softener? Is it really better to have 300 percent of the recommended daily allowance? Prenatal vitamins normally contain a daily dose of:

Folic acid (600 mcg), for prevention of birth defects
Calcium (250 mg), for bones and teeth
Choline (450 mg), for brain development
DHA (200 mg), for brain development
Iodine (250 mcg), for brain development
Iron (20–40 mg), to prevent anemia in the mother
Vitamin D (600 IU), for bones, teeth, and hormone production

The impetus to recommend prenatal vitamins began in the 1970s, when doctors discovered the relationship between low folic acid levels, found in 15 percent of women, and such birth defects as spina bifida and cleft lip. Now, nearly every pregnancy website and medical committee advises that women who are planning for pregnancy or who are pregnant should take 600 mcg of folic acid (the synthetic form of folate) per day to reduce the risk of these birth defects. Folate, also known as vitamin B$_9$, is found naturally in beans (kidney, black, lima); lentils; dark leafy greens (such as spinach), asparagus, avocados, and broccoli; tropical fruits, including mangoes, papayas, and oranges; and bread. Since 1998, the FDA has mandated that US grains, flour, and cereals be fortified with folic acid. Today, folic acid deficiency is extremely rare, affecting less than 1 percent of the US population, yet the recommendation for the supplement remains.

To decide whether you need a vitamin, you first must be honest about your diet. If vegetables and unprocessed foods never make it onto your plate, or you have dietary restrictions, a vitamin is in order. Your care provider can review your medical history and eating habits and guide you to an appropriate supplement.

the doctor's diary

I have a confession to make. I never took prenatal vitamins when I was pregnant with my kids. Not a single one. Many of my obstetrical colleagues don't take them, either. So, why do I tell my patients to use them? Because it's the norm, the recommendation of the powers that be in obstetrics, and it's the way things have always been done. Women expect to be given a prescription for vitamins, so I, like many other ob-gyns, comply. It gives women peace of mind that they are getting everything they need. Frankly, it can't hurt, but it doesn't help as much as is perceived.

VERY EXPENSIVE URINE

At $75 to $100 for a month's supply, prescription prenatal vitamins are a $3 billion industry in the United States. A vitamin requires a prescription if its amount exceeds a limit established by the FDA. For example, an over-the-counter (OTC) vitamin contains 600 mcg of folic acid, while the prescription version has 1,000 mcg. However, there is no evidence that exceeding the OTC vitamin limits makes you or your baby healthier.

the doctor's diary

I believe that prescription vitamins are a gimmick. They are expensive and rarely offer any benefits over regular vitamins. Many insurance plans don't cover them and patients, feeling that somehow these vitamins are "better," are stuck with the out-of-pocket costs.

Representatives from the vitamin manufacturers are in our offices every week, bringing lunch and samples, trying to convince us that their vitamin is better than those of their competitors. They even go so far as to have preprinted prescription pads made up with the doctor's name and the name of their vitamin, so all the doctor has to do is sign it.

Behind closed doors, physicians joke that vitamins are the ingredients in really expensive urine. So, don't feel bad if you have missed taking your vitamin or haven't taken them at all. If your doctor hands you a prescription, feel free to ask him whether there is a specific reason that you need it or whether an over-the-counter vitamin would be sufficient, and in what daily dosage.

Get Moving

Giving birth is one of the most challenging physical events you will take part in during your lifetime, and exercise during pregnancy is the best way to prepare your body for it. If you have been exercising before becoming pregnant, you can continue with that regimen as long as you feel well and have no complications. If you haven't been exercising regularly, your health and that of your baby are the perfect incentives to get you going. You can exercise right up until labor starts.

the doctor's diary

My patient Sarah has been an avid runner for many years. She took up the hobby after college as an easy way to stay fit. She wasn't breaking any records, but kept a consistent program of running about 25 miles per week. Sarah asked me how she would need to modify her routine once she was pregnant. I gave her the green light to continue with her current regimen, as long as everything was going smoothly.

Sarah signed up for a half-marathon that would take place when she was thirty weeks pregnant. She ran short distances nearly every day to prepare, and felt great. On the day of the race, it was quite warm, so she decided to run in a tank top and shorts, clearly revealing her pregnancy. She ran a few miles, walked another, and then ran again. She happily finished the race in 2:30. Much to her dismay, she received a number of dirty looks from people on the sidelines. One woman even came up to her after the race to tell her that running in pregnancy is dangerous, and that she was being selfish by competing.

Disheartened, Sarah asked me at her next office visit whether she had done something wrong. I assured her that her baby was healthy and that her fitness would surely serve her well during her upcoming labor.

Sadly, many stories appear in the media shaming pregnant women for exercising vigorously. Weight lifter Lee-Ann Ellison posted on Facebook about her achievement of lifting 75 pounds and received twenty thousand comments—many of them scolding her for doing something they believed was a risk to her pregnancy. Amber Miller completed the Chicago Marathon right before giving birth—and was upbraided by a pediatrician for having participated. Instead of making women feel guilty for staying in shape, we need to shift the focus to those pregnant women who don't exercise at all and encourage them to do so. While it may be possible to exercise to the point of injury or exhaustion, most people do not push themselves to these extremes. In nearly all cases, exercise during pregnancy is beneficial to both mom and baby.

Benefits of Exercise

Thanks to research over the last few decades, fitness professionals, doctors, and pregnant women are understanding the benefits of exercise. But many women (and their families) still believe it's harmful to break a sweat during pregnancy. Their family and friends tell them to "take it easy" and the women comply. Pregnant women tend to be less active than nonpregnant women, and due to weight gain and fatigue, their activity levels decline over the course of the pregnancy. Only 16 percent of pregnant women exercise as recommended.[8]

Until recently, doctors warned patients not to start a new exercise program or to overdo it. They insisted that women keep their heart rate below 140 beats per minute, cautioned them about overheating, and suggested that excessive exercise could prevent their baby from growing. But it turns out that none of those recommendations has science to back it up. Instead, numerous studies have proven that exercise does not hurt your baby. Blood flow to the fetus during moderate and vigorous exercise is not compromised. Exercise does not cause miscarriage, preterm labor, or small babies. You do not need to maintain your heart rate below any certain limit. Strenuous exercise is tolerated equally by the fetuses of moms who were active before pregnancy and of moms who were sedentary.

In addition to improving your overall fitness, exercising during pregnancy decreases the risk of needing a C-section by 15 percent and the chance of having an overly large baby by 25 percent. It prevents excessive weight gain, reduces low back pain, and decreases the chance of developing gestational diabetes. But despite the growing body of evidence of its benefits, the majority of ob-gyns still don't encourage their patients to exercise vigorously.

When You Shouldn't Exercise

Without a doubt, exercise is beneficial, but if you have any of the following conditions, you should not engage in an exercise routine.

- Heart disease
- Severe asthma
- Severe anemia
- Heavy smoker
- Cervical incompetence
- Persistent bleeding
- Placenta previa
- Preeclampsia
- Preterm labor

Types of Exercise

Every woman can find some type of exercise that suits her ability, preferences, and lifestyle. You should include cardiovascular, strength, and flexibility training.

At least thirty minutes of moderate cardiovascular exercise five to six days per week is recommended. This can be achieved in a variety of ways, with or without gym equipment:

- Treadmill: Run or walk, and increase the incline to increase the intensity.
- Elliptical: This machine puts less stress on the joints than running. The intensity of the workout can be easily adjusted.
- Stationary bike: Bikes also put less stress on joints, and using a stationary bike avoids issues with balance.
- Running: Jogging and running can be continued throughout pregnancy.
- Swimming: Swimming offers cardiovascular endurance without applying force to the joints.
- Walking: Walking is the most common form of exercise during pregnancy. It requires no equipment and can be done on your own schedule.

Strength training includes weight lifting and resistance exercises, such as abdominal crunches and pull-ups, which make muscles larger and stronger. Strengthening your core muscles with crunches prevents back pain and the unwanted separation of abdominal muscles called diastasis. Strong core muscles are integral to having a vaginal delivery because they provide the strength with which you will push the baby out. When working with weights during pregnancy, it is important to maintain correct alignment to protect your extra-flexible joints. How much weight is safe to lift has not been specifically determined. Working with a fitness trainer who is familiar with exercise during pregnancy can be beneficial.

Maintaining flexibility also helps you prepare for birth. Practicing yoga and Pilates is an excellent way to elongate ligaments and muscles gently and to release any tightness in the pelvis. Squatting or sitting on a chair with your legs apart has a similar effect.

Despite warnings in pregnancy books, lying flat on your back during exercising (and sleeping) is perfectly safe. This cautionary advice was based on the theory that the pregnant uterus can compress the vena cava, the large vein that runs through the abdomen, and decrease the blood flow to the baby. However, only 2 percent of women have any significant compression of this vein when lying flat, and that even with compression, the fetus is completely unaffected. If lying on your back is uncomfortable because you feel short of breath, you should move to a different position.

When to Discontinue Exercise

If you experience any of the following symptoms while exercising, you should stop immediately and contact your health-care provider.

- Bleeding
- Chest pain
- Dizziness
- Decreased fetal movement
- Preterm labor

Exercises and Activities That Should Be Avoided

Although most forms of exercise are safe, there are a few activities you should avoid while you are pregnant.

- Contact sports, such as hockey, soccer, or basketball
- Horseback riding, skiing, gymnastics, and outdoor biking have the risk that you could lose your balance and fall.
- Scuba diving

In addition, sitting or standing motionless for an extended period of time is not recommended because it impairs blood flow in the legs, which can lead to the formation of blood clots and varicose veins. If you are on a plane, road trip, or at work, you should walk every one to two hours to stimulate your circulation.

"Drink eight glasses of water per day." I see this recommendation everywhere, but it turns out it is based on no medical evidence whatsoever!

First, how much water you need depends on your weight and activity level. Second, over half of your daily water intake comes from food. Nonstarchy vegetables, such as tomatoes, cucumbers, and zucchini, are over 95 percent water. Fresh fruit contains 90 percent and even lean meats are 65 percent water. That means that your intake of drinking water—which actually means all liquids, including juice or milk—needs to be just a few glasses.

Another common myth is that, by the time you feel thirsty, you are already dehydrated. Your body is designed to send the signal of thirst well before you are in danger of dehydration. You will know that you are dehydrated if you feel dizzy and lethargic. Another good test is the color of your urine. If it is a deep yellow or orange, you need to drink more fluids. The only pregnant women who are truly at risk of dehydration are those with severe vomiting or diarrhea.

You can stop carrying around the water bottle at all times and just drink when you feel thirsty.

Strong Abs + Relaxed Vagina = Easy Delivery

The ability of a baby to maneuver through the birth canal to the outside world relies on the strength of the muscles pushing it out and the stretching of the muscles holding it in. Uterine contractions and your abdominal muscles provide the downward forces as the tightness of your pelvic floor and vaginal muscles releases. Having strong core muscles and loose vaginal muscles is the best way to ensure an easy delivery.

To prepare your vaginal muscles for childbirth, you want them to be as stretchy as possible, especially at the opening. Massaging the perineum (the muscles between the vaginal opening and the anus) during the last six weeks of pregnancy decreases the chance of tearing.

How to massage the perineum: Put two fingers inside the vaginal opening and apply pressure straight downward for two minutes, then apply pressure to each side for two minutes. This massage should be done daily with a lubricant from thirty-four weeks until delivery.

Kegel exercises strengthen the pelvic floor muscles, and have the opposite effect of perineal massage. While massage makes the muscles looser, Kegels makes them tighter. Performing Kegel exercises will not make your birth easier or decrease your risk of tearing. Women with extremely strong pelvic floor muscles have more resistance to the baby coming out. Therefore, Kegel exercises should only be used during pregnancy to combat urinary incontinence. They can be used in the postpartum period to counter pelvic organ prolapse.

Causes and Prevention of Birth Defects

Birth defects occur in 3 percent of all pregnancies. Some birth defects are minor, whereas others lead to serious health issues and disabilities. Birth defects originate from infections, exposure to toxins, genetic mutations, and maternal medical conditions, but for the majority, the cause is unknown. Most defects develop in the first trimester when the fetus's organs are forming, affecting how the baby looks or how its body functions.

Mothers at the extremes of age have a greater chance of having a baby with a birth defect. Babies born to teenagers have a higher incidence of structural abnormalities, including anencephaly (absence of the brain), hydrocephaly (excess fluid around the brain), extra fingers, gastroschisis (when the intestines are outside the body), or cleft lip and palate. Mothers over age thirty-five have an increased risk of having babies with chromosomal birth defects, such as Down syndrome. Overall, women aged twenty-five to thirty have the lowest risk.

Genetic problems, such as gene mutations, extra or missing chromosomes, and genes that do not work properly, cannot be prevented. These problems are related to the age of the mother, are inherited, or can occur spontaneously.

AUTISM SPECTRUM DISORDERS

Autism is not a birth defect but it is one of the conditions pregnant women worry about most. What can they do to prevent their baby from having this? Autism is a developmental disability that affects communication and interaction with others. Some children with autism speak very little, obsessively focus on one interest, and have problems reading social cues, such as facial expressions and gestures. The autistic spectrum includes a wide array of disorders where some are only mildly affected, whereas others cannot have any normal social interactions without relentless intervention and are unable to live independently. Some people with autism spectrum disorder excel in art, math, and music.

In the United States, 1 in 88 children has an autism spectrum disorder (1 in 31 boys, 1 in 143 girls). During the 1970s and 1980s, the incidence was only 1 in 2,000, leading scientists to wonder if autism is on the rise, or simply detected more frequently—particularly among children who are relatively high functioning. If autism is on the rise, why so?

While speculation is rampant on this topic, the cause of autism is still unknown. Most likely, it results from an interaction between genes and environmental exposures. Scientists have identified changes in the fetal brain, particularly in the outer layers responsible for language, which are linked to autism, thereby concluding that the disorder begins during pregnancy. Early intervention in toddlers, such as strategies to promote communication, may rewire some of these areas of the brain that have developed abnormally.

Autism occurs more frequently in children of older mothers, older fathers, mothers with gestational diabetes and preexisting diabetes, and those who have used certain medications like antidepressants. It is also linked to low-birth-weight babies, being born in March or April, having fetal distress during labor or a birth injury, and passing meconium.

Environmental causes: Women who live in areas with high levels of pollution—involving toxins from lead, manganese, and methylene chloride—are 50 percent more likely to have a child with autism. Pesticides and polychlorinated biphenyls (PCBs) may also be contributing factors. Although PCBs—chemicals used in electrical equipment and fluorescent lighting—were banned in the United States in 1979, they may still linger in the environment.

Genetic causes: A few hundred different genes have been associated with autism. If one identical twin is autistic, there is 75 percent chance the other will be affected. In addition, certain genes may cause a child to be more susceptible to environmental factors.

Avoiding Birth Defects

Every mother wants to do what she can to ensure that her baby develops normally. Things you can do prior to, and during, your pregnancy to prevent birth defects include:

- Take a folic acid supplement if your diet lacks it. Folic acid decreases the risk of neural tube defects (NTD) by 90 percent if consumed during first 28 days of pregnancy. It is found in enriched grain products, such as rice, cereal, bread, and pasta; green vegetables; and beans as well as vitamin supplements.[9]
- Be evaluated for diabetes. High blood sugar during pregnancy causes heart defects.
- Maintain a healthy weight. Obesity increases the risk of numerous birth defects, such as spina bifida, heart defects, cleft lip, and hydrocephaly.
- Avoid fevers/flu. Having a fever over 101 degrees Fahrenheit during the first trimester increases the risk of heart defects and spina bifida. Acetaminophen can be used safely to bring down a fever. Pregnant women can protect

themselves by being vaccinated against the flu, washing
their hands regularly, and avoiding close contact with anyone who is sick.

- Avoid alcohol. Excessive consumption of alcohol during
  pregnancy causes fetal alcohol syndrome, which is char-
  acterized by an abnormal facial structure, hyperactivity,
  impaired motor skills, and intellectual disability.
- Stop smoking. Nicotine causes poor fetal growth, stillbirth,
  and cleft lip.
- Prevent infection by *Toxoplasma*, cytomegalovirus (CMV),
  Listeria, chickenpox, and rubella.
  - Heat all meats before eating. This includes hot dogs,
    deli meats, and steak.
  - Avoid saliva from children, including your own. Don't
    put your child's toothbrush, pacifier, or utensils in
    your mouth or kiss children on the mouth.
  - Wash your hands thoroughly with soap and water
    after handling raw meats or after changing diapers,
    feeding a child, or wiping a child's nose.
  - See "Understanding Infections," page 54, for more
    about specific infections.
- Confirm with your doctor whether your prescription
  and over-the-counter medications are safe for use during
  pregnancy.
- Try to avoid known environmental toxins in your home
  and work.

Vices: The Truth About Cannabis, Alcohol, Caffeine, and Tobacco

Prior to the 1970s, pregnant women regularly enjoyed a cocktail
and a cigarette after dinner. Times have certainly changed, as we
now know much more about the impact that alcohol, cigarettes, and
recreational drugs have on a pregnant woman and, in turn, on her
growing fetus.

Cannabis: Two to 5 percent of pregnant women use marijuana. Despite its prevalence and its legalization for medical and recreational use in several US states, there are no conclusive studies about its safety during pregnancy. Many users are also more likely to smoke cigarettes, drink alcohol, use other drugs, and have poor nutrition.

Marijuana has been used as medicine for thousands of years, with its effects documented back to the seventh century. It can treat nausea, glaucoma, seizures, anxiety, and pain. Tetrahydrocannabinol (THC), its active ingredient, crosses the placenta and appears in fetal blood at 10 percent of maternal levels. Studies have shown that cannabis does not cause preterm delivery or birth defects and does not affect the baby's birth weight or the overall pregnancy outcome. Research on children's development, including verbal reasoning, memory, attention span, and behavioral changes, is inconclusive.

Despite a lack of concrete evidence that marijuana is dangerous, the American College of Obstetricians and Gynecologists (ACOG) recommends that women should not use it while pregnant.

Alcohol: Although socially acceptable and legal, alcohol is the drug with the greatest impact on the physical and mental development of a child. There is no known amount of alcohol that is proven safe in pregnancy.

Alcohol can cause fetal alcohol syndrome (FAS), the leading cause of mental disability in the world. Affecting 1 in 500 children, this condition permanently damages a baby. Common characteristics are abnormal facial features, a small head, short stature, intellectual impairment, learning disabilities, and a low IQ. FAS develops in 3 percent of babies whose mothers consumed at least six drinks per day. Clearly, heavy drinking is dangerous.

Conclusions about drinking small amounts of alcohol are harder to come by. Of course, scientists can't force women to drink certain amounts of alcohol to see how it affects their babies. In addition, women who are asked to recall how much they drank at different times during pregnancy may underreport what actually happened. Keep in mind that there are also genetic differences in the ability to metabolize alcohol and the same amount of alcohol may affect different women in dissimilar ways.

Observations about the effects of alcohol vary significantly from one study to another. One shows that eight drinks per week doesn't cause any problems, while the next suggests that only one drink per week may impact fetal growth.

So, what should you do? Can you have a glass of wine with dinner? Interestingly, many women describe a change in the taste of alcohol when they are pregnant, making it naturally less desirable. Having a drink or two occasionally is probably fine, but you shouldn't make it a regular occurrence.

Caffeine is one of the most commonly used and highly addictive drugs in the United States, with over 80 percent of adults consuming it daily. Caffeine increases alertness, elevates stress hormone levels, and raises the heart rate. Withdrawal symptoms include headaches, irritability, and nausea. Caffeine can be safely consumed during pregnancy as it does not cause miscarriage, preterm birth, poor fetal growth, or birth defects. Even with no evidence that it is harmful, most public health authorities suggest that pregnant women limit caffeine intake to 200 to 300 mg per day, the equivalent of one or two cups of coffee.

the doctor's diary

How did coffee become a no-no in pregnancy? Scientists observed that women who miscarry tend to drink more coffee than do women who carry the pregnancy to term. They concluded that caffeine may be a cause of miscarriage.

It turns out that the difference in coffee drinking habits has to do with food aversions in the first trimester. Women with healthy pregnancies tend to dislike certain foods and strong odors and instinctively avoid things like coffee. Women with nonviable pregnancies (destined to miscarry) don't feel as "pregnant" and are more likely to eat and drink as usual.

Of course, many women with normal pregnancies don't have aversions to coffee, so you shouldn't use your caffeine cravings to gauge the health of your pregnancy.

Caffeine doesn't cause miscarriage, but these past theories live on as many organizations still recommend limiting its intake, without science to back it up.

Smoking cigarettes negatively affects your health and that of your baby. Nicotine causes blood vessels to constrict, significantly decreasing the flow of oxygen to the fetus. Smoking has been proven to cause miscarriage, poor fetal growth, birth defects, and preterm delivery. The effect is seen even in light smokers who consume fewer than ten cigarettes per day. Despite the warnings about the dangers of tobacco use, 10 percent of pregnant women still smoke. Even secondhand smoke has its dangers, including poor fetal growth and sudden infant death syndrome (SIDS).

Nicotine gums and patches have the same effect of decreasing the blood flow, but they do not contain any of the other five hundred carcinogens that are found in tobacco, such as tar, ammonia, benzene, and carbon monoxide. Similarly, e-cigarettes (electronic nicotine delivery systems) contain nicotine just like regular cigarettes, without the additional toxins in smoke.

Attitudes about smoking during pregnancy have changed dramatically over the last fifty years. A print ad for Winston cigarettes in the 1950s featured a picture of a pregnant woman with a cigarette and the caption: "Taste isn't the only reason I smoke. People are always telling me that smoking causes low birth weight. Talk about a win-win-win! An easy labor, a slim baby, and the full flavor of Winstons!" It concludes with: "Winston: When You Are Smoking for Two." Contrary to the wisdom of the Winston ads, if a baby is small because of low oxygen levels during pregnancy, the child may have other health issues later in life, including cerebral palsy, learning problems, and chronic infections.

If You Drank Alcohol or Smoked Before You Knew You Were Pregnant

Because half of all pregnancies are unplanned, there are bound to be many women who were drinking alcohol, smoking, or using other drugs before they knew they were pregnant. They feel panicked that the pregnancy they didn't plan but truly want may be affected by their actions. The developing embryo is particularly sensitive to toxins, called teratogens, from the time of conception to the time of implantation, which occurs five days later. The effect of a teratogen during this short window follows the "all or none" rule. If an exposure was severely toxic, the pregnancy will miscarry. If the embryo continues to grow, it means that the toxin did not have any effect.

Exposure to teratogens from eighteen to sixty days after conception (gestational age 4 ½ to 10 ½ weeks) is most likely to cause birth defects. During this time, the fetal organs are developing rapidly and damage to them cannot be repaired. Typically, a urine pregnancy test will be positive twelve days after conception and a woman will miss her period fourteen days after conception. Therefore, once you find out you are pregnant, you should avoid unnecessary exposures during these critical weeks.

Understanding Infections

Viruses and bacterial infections can range from unpleasant to debilitating. When you are pregnant, some of them can also affect your unborn child.

Cytomegalovirus (CMV)

Incidence: CMV is the most common viral infection that affects fetuses. One in every 150 babies in the United States is born with congenital CMV (about 30,000 children per year).

Symptoms: Fever, fatigue, muscle aches, sore throat.

How it is transmitted: CMV is found in bodily fluids, such as blood, saliva, urine, and tears. It is most commonly spread from a child to an adult through close contact and kissing.

Effect on developing fetus: Congenital CMV causes blindness, deafness, seizures, and/or mental disabilities in the newborn.

Detection: A blood test can show whether you have been exposed in the past (and are immune to CMV) or whether you have had a recent exposure.

Treatment: None.

Prevention: Women should wash their hands after feeding children, wiping a child's nose, or handling toys. Do not share food, drinks, or utensils with, and avoid kisses from, children.

Listeria

Incidence: There are 1,600 infections from *Listeria* per year in the United States, affecting 225 pregnant women. Some recent outbreaks: in 2015, Blue Bell ice cream; 2015, Granny Smith apples; 2014, caramel apples; 2014, sprouts; 2011, cantaloupes; and 2005, turkey deli meat.

Symptoms: Fever, muscle aches, stiff neck.

How it is transmitted: Listeria is a bacteria found in soil, uncooked meats, vegetables, unpasteurized milk and cheese, and processed foods (deli meats, smoked seafood). The bacteria can be killed by heating food and pasteurization.

Effect on developing fetus: If a woman has listeriosis during pregnancy, there is a 90 percent chance that she will pass it to the fetus. *Listeria* can cause miscarriage, stillbirth (occurs in 20 percent of babies who were exposed), and preterm labor.

Detection: Blood culture.

Treatment: Antibiotics.

Prevention: Avoid unpasteurized cheeses, such as feta, Brie, and Camembert. Cook meats and reheat leftover foods thoroughly.

Rinse raw produce. Do not eat hot dogs or deli meats unless they are heated to 165 degrees Fahrenheit. Do not eat pâté or meat spread. Avoid smoked seafood unless it is cooked or canned.

Rubella (German measles)

Incidence: The Western Hemisphere became the world's first region to eliminate rubella and congenital rubella syndrome in 2015 through extensive vaccination programs. In other parts of the world, rubella continues to affect over 100,000 newborns per year.

Symptoms: Rash and fever.

How it is transmitted: Coughing and sneezing.

Effect on developing fetus: Congenital rubella syndrome causes deafness, cataracts, heart defects, intellectual disability, miscarriage, and stillbirth.

Detection: Observation of the rash, confirmed with blood tests.

Treatment: None.

Prevention: Vaccination prior to pregnancy.

Toxoplasma

Incidence: Forty percent of the US population is immune to toxoplasma because of a previous exposure. There are four hundred to eight hundred cases of fetal infection per year.

Symptoms: Can be asymptomatic or involve body aches, fever, and fatigue.

How it is transmitted: Nearly all cases of toxoplasmosis are from consuming raw or undercooked meat. It can spread from contaminated knives and cutting boards. Despite numerous pregnancy websites' suggesting that women should never change a litter box or pet a cat during pregnancy, cats are an extremely rare source of this infection. The parasite can be passed in the feces of cats who have contracted it from eating garbage. Women are then exposed if they touch their mouths after handling the cat's feces, which, thankfully, doesn't happen often. It happens even less, or never, when the cats in your life are well-fed pets kept exclusively indoors.

Effect on developing fetus: Congenital toxoplasmosis causes blindness, seizures, jaundice, and intellectual disability.

Detection: Blood test to look for antibodies to the parasite.

Treatment: Antibiotics.

Prevention: Keep your cat indoors and feed it dry or canned cat food, instead of raw meat. If your cat goes outdoors, have someone else clean the litter box. Wear gloves when gardening. Wash your hands, knives, and cutting boards thoroughly when handling raw meats. Cook meats thoroughly. Wash all produce.

Varicella (chicken pox)

Incidence: Varicella affects 400 to 800 babies per year.

Symptoms: Itchy rash, pneumonia, fevers, malaise.

How it is transmitted: Chicken pox, also known as human herpesvirus 3, is spread from person to person through coughing and sneezing.

Effect on developing fetus: Congenital varicella syndrome causes scars on fetal skin, low birth weight, and nervous system abnormalities.

Detection: Observation of rash; confirmed through blood tests.

Treatment: Antiviral medication, such as acyclovir or valacyclovir.

Prevention: Varicella vaccine can be given prior to pregnancy. Avoid contact with people sick with chicken pox. If a nonimmune pregnant woman is exposed to someone with the chicken pox, she should receive varicella zoster immunoglobulin (VZIG).

Zika Virus

Incidence: As of June 2016, about a thousand cases of Zika were reported in the United States.

Symptoms: Most people with Zika have no symptoms, but 30 percent will develop fever, rash, red eyes, and joint pain. Symptoms last for one week after infection.

How it is transmitted: Zika is spread through bites from the Aedes mosquito, but it can also pass between sexual partners.

Effect on developing fetus: If a pregnant woman gets Zika, she can pass it to her fetus, causing severe birth defects, such as microcephaly (abnormally small head and brain), as well as deafness, blindness, seizures and difficulty swallowing.

Detection: Zika virus testing can be done through a blood test. Testing should be done for any woman who is pregnant and has traveled to an area where there has been a Zika outbreak.

Treatment: There is no treatment yet available.

Prevention: Avoid travel to areas where the virus is prevalent if you are pregnant or trying to become pregnant. If you are in a Zika area, use insect repellent. Repellents with at least 7 percent DEET or 20 percent picaridin are the most effective against Aedes mosquitos and are considered safe during pregnancy. Wear long-sleeved shirts and long pants. Check that enclosures, such as screened porches, are free of holes. Eliminate standing water.

Use condoms for six months if your partner has been to an area with Zika. Women should wait eight weeks before attempting pregnancy if they have traveled to an area with Zika.

Environmental Exposures

The incidence of childhood leukemia has increased 20 percent in the last two decades. Autism has seen a rise of 600 percent. There is a fourfold increase in asthma. Attention-deficit disorder (ADD) has increased 40 percent. Although the direct cause has not been proven, some of these increases may be the result of exposure to toxins in our environment, such as air pollution, industrial chemicals, and pesticides.[10]

Despite a growing body of anecdotal and preliminary evidence that environmental exposures may significantly impact pregnant women and their babies, ob-gyns rarely—only 20 percent in a recent survey—discuss this issue with their patients. Doctors refrain from this conversation because of a lack of concrete evidence about the consequences of exposures. In addition, mentioning every exposure that could be potentially harmful may overwhelm a patient and cause confusion and anxiety.

Such organizations as ACOG and the FDA assert that there is not enough information to determine exactly which exposures are dangerous. Doctors, scientists, and consumers attempt to rate the relative safety of chemical compounds in our environment. Ideally, the burden of proof should lie with chemical companies themselves. However, studies are limited because pregnant women can't knowingly be exposed by researchers to something that is potentially harmful. In addition, the majority of chemicals produced in the United States have never been tested for safety in animals or humans because the Environmental Protection Agency does not require it.

Air Pollution

Air pollution is caused by excessive amounts of carbon monoxide, sulfur dioxide, ammonia, and nitrogen dioxide. These substances are produced in manufacturing plants and from burning coal and gasoline. Air pollution is linked to higher rates of preterm delivery, poor fetal growth, and lung problems in newborns. Its negative impact on children is especially noticeable for families who live near steel mills, oil refineries, and chemical treatment plants, as well as in areas with high industrial and automotive emissions.

Pregnant women who live in an area with high pollution or near a freeway should consider purchasing a HEPA (high-efficiency particulate absorption) filter for their homes. These filters eliminate over 99 percent of pollution from the air. While their use has not specifically been shown to improve birth outcomes, they are certainly beneficial for adults with asthma or allergies.

Atrazine

The herbicide atrazine is used to prevent weeds from growing within corn crops. Three quarters of all US corn is treated with atrazine. It is used on golf courses and Christmas tree lots, and can be found in local water supplies, especially in farming communities of the Midwest. Atrazine, banned in Europe since 2003, converts testosterone to estrogen in the human body and has been linked to poor fetal growth and prematurity. Studies on atrazine exposure in humans are limited and no definitive conclusions can be made.

To avoid atrazine exposure during pregnancy, buy organic produce. Using a carbon water filter in your home is effective at removing atrazine from tap water.

Bisphenol A

Bisphenol A (BPA), a chemical used to harden plastics, is found in the liners of canned foods, water bottles, paper receipts, and eyeglasses. It enters our body through food that was in containers made with BPA. It can disrupt hormone levels in the developing fetus, affect behavior in children, and could potentially be linked to cancer, diabetes, and heart disease in adults.

One study of umbilical cord blood found BPA present in 100 percent of newborns. The FDA says that BPA is safe at the current levels. However, reducing exposure to BPA could be beneficial. Plastics labeled "BPA-free" often contain alternatives, such as bisphenol S, which may have effects similar to those of BPA. During pregnancy, you should replace plastic with glass or stainless-steel containers.

Lead

Lead is toxic to the nervous system of the developing fetus and has been linked to miscarriage, poor fetal growth, and lower IQ. It was banned from gasoline in 1973 and was removed from residential paint and plumbing in 1978. However, lead can still be found in deteriorating paint (dust and paint chips) and pipes in older homes. If you are remodeling a house painted prior to 1978, the paint dust and any debris must be removed by a licensed contractor to reduce lead contamination.

Women of childbearing age may still have lead in their systems from exposure as children or from lead pipes. If you live in an older home, or if you don't know what kind of plumbing you have, you can ask your doctor to check your lead level. Lead continues to be stored in our bones for many years after exposure. During pregnancy, as calcium is mobilized from bones, lead can leak into the bloodstream as well. Taking calcium supplements during pregnancy will prevent your bones from releasing these lead stores.

Mercury

This chemical occurs naturally in the air and is also a by-product of industrial pollution. When it falls into water, it turns into methyl mercury, which can build up in fish—especially tilefish, shark, swordfish, and king mackerel. Infants of mothers with high mercury levels have a lower IQ, intellectual disability, difficulty with movement, blindness, and seizures.

Pesticides

All pesticides pose some risk during pregnancy. Nearly all people carry pesticide residue in their body from the foods they eat, exposures in gardens and yards, and the use of insecticides in the home. Women with higher pesticide concentrations give birth to smaller babies. These children are more likely to develop attention-deficit/hyperactivity disorder (ADHD), learning problems, and a lower IQ.

Produce that is grown above the ground has the highest pesticide residue, whereas root vegetables, vegetables with a husk, and fruits with a thick, inedible rind have the least. High levels are seen in green beans, peppers, spinach, pears, peaches, and apples. To reduce pesticide exposure, you should wash all produce with a brush to remove the residue. If it is not cost-prohibitive, eating organic produce eliminates exposure because it is pesticide-free.

Phthalates

Phthalates are chemicals that make plastics softer and more flexible. They are found in hundreds of products, including IV bags and tubing, plastic wrap, shampoo, shower curtains, raincoats, nail polish, children's toys, and plastic food containers. A 2010 study suggested that exposure to phthalates during pregnancy lowered testosterone levels in boys, leading to changes in the shape of their genitals and less male-typical play behavior.[11] Needless to say, this study started a panic among pregnant women as well as officials at the Environmental Protection Agency, which chose to ban the substance from children's toys. Hundreds of studies on phthalates have since failed to support the original findings.

By far, the most common source of phthalates is plastic food storage containers, plastic-lined cans, and plastic wrap. To be safe during pregnancy, you can limit your use of these products.

Sweeteners

Nutritive sweeteners (table sugar, honey, fructose, maltose, and dextrose) add sweet flavor and calories, but contain few vitamins or minerals. They are safe in pregnancy.

Nonnutritive sweeteners are calorie-free and are generally safe:

Stevia: Safe
Aspartame (Equal and NutraSweet): Safe
Sucralose (Splenda): Safe
Saccharine (Sweet'N Low): Unknown

Workplace Exposures

A National Health and Nutrition Examination Survey done in 2004 found that every pregnant woman of the 268 tested had at least forty-three different chemicals in her blood.[12] Many exposures occur in the workplace. Here are some areas of employment and their risks for exposure:

Artists: Solvents and heavy metals, such as lead.
Childcare workers: CMV, chicken pox.

Dry cleaning: Perchloroethylene (solvent used in dry cleaning). Exposure to this solvent is not significant for women wearing clothes that have been dry-cleaned, but there may be a risk of miscarriage for women working with the solvent regularly.

Farmworkers: Pesticides such as ethylene dibromide and atrazine.

Hairdressers/nail salons: Chemical solvents has been linked to some birth defects, but have not been seen in women who have their hair dyed or nails painted.

Health-care workers: Hydrogen peroxide gas, formaldehyde. It is not known what levels of these exposures are safe.

Pilots and flight attendants: Exposure to cosmic ionizing radiation.

Restaurant waitpersons/bartenders: Secondhand smoke.

Typical products that you may encounter at work that *don't* pose any harm to the fetus include ammonia, hydrochloric acid, bleach, fiberglass, and asbestos.

Home Products

Home cleaning products contain a variety of chemicals. Unfortunately, scientific studies on the safety of specific products during pregnancy are sparse. Due to ethical considerations, most research is done in animals only—with much of that now considered inhumane and being phased out—and not in humans. In addition, many products do not contain a list of ingredients because the formulations are patent-protected, making it difficult for the consumer to determine whether the product is safe.

Women who are pregnant can avoid unnecessary exposure from household products by wearing gloves and making sure the room is well ventilated when these products are used. They can clean with baking soda, lemon juice, hydrogen peroxide, and white vinegar, or buy products that contain all-natural ingredients.

Products to avoid or use with caution:

- Mildew removers
- Brass and silver polish
- Wood finish sprays
- Fragrant laundry detergents and air fresheners
- Antibacterial hand soap
- Pesticides, insecticides, and flea collars
- Floor wax and polish
- Drain cleaners

Products that are safe:

- **Paint:** Paint is now made without volatile organic compounds, so it is considered safe.
- **Nail polish:** Check to make sure it is formaldehyde- and phthalate-free.
- **Carpets and rugs:** The latex backing and the synthetic fibers in carpets and rugs emits a gas, but it is not harmful.

Medications

The FDA has recently made major changes in how prescription drugs are categorized for use in pregnancy. For every drug, there is a risk summary that describes known birth defects, and links to miscarriage or fetal growth problems. Ultimately, the decision to take a prescription drug requires an evaluation of the risks and benefits. Information can be found on the drug insert or by consulting your provider.

Medications That Should Not Be Taken During Pregnancy

Some medications are known to cause birth defects. If you are taking any medications, you should talk to your doctor about their safety during pregnancy. If your condition is mild, you may be able to discontinue the medication altogether, lower your dosage, or to switch to another medication that is safe. In some cases, you may have no choice but to continue on a medication that has risks.

- Acne treatment: Accutane
- Antibiotics: streptomycin, tetracycline
- Antidepressants: Paxil, Prozac. Paxil and Prozac, unlike other selective serotonin reuptake inhibitors (SSRIs), have been linked to certain birth defects such as anencephaly and heart problems. Pregnant women with mild depression may be able to be weaned off all antidepressants. However, those with moderate or severe depression should discontinue Paxil or Prozac and switch to another antidepressant, such as Zoloft, Celexa, or Lexapro, in consultation with their doctor.[13]
- Anxiety medication: benzodiazepines (Valium, Ativan, Xanax)
- Bipolar medication: lithium
- Blood thinner: Coumadin
- Blood pressure medicine: ACE inhibitors, thiazide diuretics (hydrochlorothiazide, Lasix)
- Cholesterol-lowering drugs: Lipitor, Crestor, Pravachol
- Live-virus vaccines: measles-mumps-rubella (MMR), varicella, yellow fever
- Seizure medication: phenobarbital, Dilantin, valproate. Women who need to take these medications should switch to something safer, such as Keppra or Lamictal, in consultation with their doctor.

Over-the-Counter Medications

Many over-the-counter (OTC) medications are safe in pregnancy, including Tylenol (acetaminophen), Benadryl (diphenhydramine), Claritin (loratidine), Sudafed (pseudoephedrine), cough medicines, Colace, Metamucil, Milk of Magnesia, Tums, Pepcid, and Zantac.

The few OTC medications that should be avoided are aspirin at high doses, ibuprofen (Motrin, Advil), and naproxen (Aleve).

Herbal Remedies

The FDA doesn't evaluate herbs or homeopathic treatments for safety or efficacy. Therefore, it may be prudent to avoid these, especially during the first trimester.

Herbs that shouldn't be taken by pregnant women:

- Black cohosh
- Blue cohosh
- Chasteberry
- Dong quai
- Garlic
- Gingko
- Ginseng
- Mugwort
- Red clover
- St. John's wort
- Saw palmetto
- Valerian
- Wormwood

Supplements that have *not* been linked to any poor outcomes in pregnancy are:

- Cranberry
- Chamomile
- Echinacea
- Fish oil
- Ginger

Information about the dos and don'ts during pregnancy may seem daunting. Faced with the advice of your sister, the guidance of your doctor, and the litany of "facts" on the Internet, you may feel like you need to protect yourself from everything. The truth is that much of taking care of yourself in pregnancy is common sense. Plenty of healthy babies have been born to mothers who had a glass of wine, ate salami, and played with their cats. Most things that are dangerous require chronic exposure over the course of the pregnancy. It's important not to get stressed about the small details, such as whether it's safe to wear nail polish or have a cup of coffee. Most likely, you won't find these guidelines difficult to follow or the sacrifices too great. Instead, you will feel good about taking control of your pregnancy and health.

CHOOSING WHO, WHERE, AND HOW

—from MDs to Midwives, Hospitals to Home

Nothing influences your experience of pregnancy and childbirth as much as whom you choose as your health-care provider, where you plan to give birth, and how you prepare for the occasion. Both doctors and midwives are trained to deliver babies. However, their philosophies may be worlds apart. Giving birth in your own home can feel comfortable and familiar; giving birth in a hospital can feel safe and protected in case of an emergency. Understanding the differences between the myriad of options available will allow you to choose the best fit for you and your baby.

Doctors and Midwives—What's the Difference?

Physicians view birth as a medical process with well-defined risks that can be reduced with interventions. Midwives take a more holistic approach, viewing birth as a natural experience and intervening only when necessary. A doctor *delivers* your baby and a midwife *attends* your birth. If your labor stalls, a doctor will help get the baby out. A midwife will guide you in what you need to do to birth your baby. You can choose a doctor or midwife, but you generally do not need both.

the doctor's diary

When there is a plane crash, one of the first things reported in the news is how many hours of flying time the pilot had in that particular aircraft. The more time spent, the more likely the pilot could handle an emergency. The same is true in obstetrics—the more experience, the better. I had delivered more than one thousand babies before I experienced my first uterine inversion (where a uterus turns inside out after delivery), a rare obstetrical emergency. As an OB resident, I was trained to manage this complication through simulated drills. But I had never seen one until I had been practicing for a number of years. In obstetrics, when things go well, a delivery is effortless. When things go badly, a small problem can steamroll into a major catastrophe within minutes. From complicated vaginal lacerations, a bleeding placenta accreta, amniotic fluid embolisms, and eclamptic seizures—I never feel like I can breathe a sigh of relief until I know the mother and baby are on their way home from the hospital safely.

The skills to handle obstetrical emergencies come from education, training, and hands-on experience. When choosing a provider, you should understand her background. If your doctor has completed an accredited residency program, most likely she has been well trained and is experienced. You can inquire how many deliveries she has attended and whether she is board certified. If you are seeing a midwife, you can ask about her education and licensure as well.

During training, a doctor will participate in hundreds of births; a student midwife, only thirty to forty. Although the doctor's numbers are higher, he may actually only be at the patient's bedside at the last moment to catch the baby. A student midwife trains in a manner that is unrushed, spending hours or days with her patient, and focusing on the subtle details of labor, instead of just the grand finale. There are benefits to both approaches.

Beware of Bias

Your provider should give you accurate and unbiased information without pushing her personal agenda. If her goal is to provide you only with a specific birth experience, she may color the conversation so you follow that path. For example, if your baby is breech, a doctor may schedule you for a cesarean without considering and discussing other options, such as trying to turn the baby. Similarly, if you are planning a home birth and your baby is breech, a midwife may insist that you can still have a vaginal birth at home, although it may in fact be dangerous, and in some states illegal to do so.

Of course, your provider will have opinions about what is best for you. But an opinion is different than a bias. Your provider may be biased if she only gives one option for a given situation, sees one side of an argument, or ignores what is important to you.

Doctors

An obstetrician-gynecologist (ob-gyn) provides prenatal care for normal healthy women, diagnoses and treats pregnancy complications, takes care of gynecologic problems, and performs pelvic surgery. The thirty-five thousand ob-gyns currently practicing in the United States deliver 92 percent of the nation's babies. An ob-gyn first receives a bachelor's degree in any area of study from a university and then attends medical school for four years. He applies for a residency position by submitting medical school grades, board exam scores, recommendations from professors, a summary of research and work experience, and then attending an interview. Residency positions are competitive, with approximately 1,800 applicants every year for 1,200 available spots. During residency, he learns obstetrics, gynecology, fertility, oncology, and other aspects of women's health care. He presents cases for discussion to his professors, attends conferences, and cares for patients. He delivers hundreds of babies, many in high-risk situations. He must pass two written national board exams.

After residency, an ob-gyn can join a private practice, teach, or work directly for a hospital. He may practice general obstetrics and gynecology or undergo additional training to become a subspecialist. There are four subspecialties in ob-gyn: oncology, maternal-fetal medicine, reproductive endocrinology, and pelvic surgery.

the doctor's diary

My patients often ask me whether I am a "high-risk" OB (someone who takes care of pregnancies with complications). Actually, managing complications is the basis of obstetrical training, so all OBs are "high-risk specialists." Being able to care for high-risk patients is not a special designation within this field.

A Doctor's Philosophy

Doctors deliver hundreds of babies during training. They witness completely normal pregnancies quickly take an unexpected turn to become high risk. They see babies get stuck on their way out, postpartum bleeding requiring an immediate hysterectomy, and young healthy women having eclamptic seizures. Doctors are trained to prepare for the worst, but hope for the best. They seek to identify complications, even before symptoms are obvious. They have the skills to provide any medical intervention necessary and feel comfortable doing so. A doctor believes that he should attend every delivery in case of an emergency.

I rarely saw a "normal" delivery when I was in my residency. Nearly every patient had some sort of intervention. When I began private practice, I was uncomfortable with the idea of a patient's having only intermittent fetal monitoring, or not having an IV during labor. Laboring without a monitor or IV is considered more "natural," and yet it took me years of experience to feel comfortable with that approach. I was so focused on looking for abnormalities, that "natural" seemed as if it were the unusual way to deliver.

Thankfully, as time went on, I was able to unwind these habits. I'm happy to help a woman have a natural birth, but am ready in the event an intervention is needed.

MD, DO, and FACOG—What the Letters Tell You About Your Doctor

When a student graduates from medical school, he is given an MD (medical doctor) or DO (doctor of osteopathy) degree. He must then complete a one-year internship program, which can be done in any field—internal medicine, pediatrics, ob-gyn, and other disciplines. At the end of this year, if he passes an exam, he can become licensed by the state in which he practices. Once licensed, he can prescribe medication, perform surgery, and give general medical care.

If the new doctor chooses to become an ob-gyn, he must complete a residency program in obstetrics and gynecology and pass a series of written and oral exams. To become board certified, the doctor then compiles a list of every patient whom he has cared for during his first two years after residency, outlining their diagnosis and treatment. This list is sent to the American Board of Obstetrics and Gynecology for review. If the list illustrates an adequate depth and breadth of knowledge, he is invited to take a day-long oral board exam administered by experts in the field. If he passes this final test, he is considered a board-certified ob-gyn and can apply to become a fellow of the American College of Obstetricians and Gynecologists (FACOG). Once certified, he must maintain this designation by completing a review of knowledge about the current medical literature annually and passing a written exam every six years.

Seventy percent of practicing ob-gyns has this certification. If your doctor is board certified, you can feel confident that she is knowledgeable and experienced in the field. Some doctors choose not to be certified because they don't have time to prepare for the exams or keep up on the current medical education. Others aren't certified because they never passed the exams. You can check the status of your doctor on the website www.abog.org.

A physician who is not board certified may be experienced and can be licensed to practice in his state. But there is no way to guarantee his skill level or the quality of care he can deliver. If your doctor isn't board certified, ask him why. If he hasn't yet been in practice for two years after residency, it may simply be because he hasn't qualified to take the test yet. In this case, the doctor is considered board eligible. If the doctor hasn't been able to pass the exams or chose not to take them, you should consider another physician.

A Perinatologist

A perinatologist is an ob-gyn who has completed an additional three years of fellowship training in the subspecialty of maternal-fetal medicine. Perinatologists are experts in ultrasound; genetic testing, such as amniocentesis and chorionic villus sampling; and management of high-risk pregnancies. Normally a perinatologist does not deliver babies but, rather, gives advice to your regular ob-gyn or midwife regarding your care and delivery. For example, a woman with high blood pressure may see a perinatologist every few weeks to evaluate the growth of the baby by ultrasound. If this doctor determines that the baby isn't growing well, she would advise your ob-gyn to induce labor, but wouldn't undertake the induction herself. Many patients see a perinatologist at least once during a pregnancy, usually at around twenty weeks, for a detailed ultrasound.

A Laborist

A laborist is an ob-gyn who cares for women during labor, and is usually employed by the hospital itself, working twelve- to twenty-four-hour shifts. Laborists do not provide prenatal care or have office responsibilities, but are available to help any patient who has an emergency if her regular doctor isn't available. Some hospitals also utilize laborists to deliver all the patients in the labor and delivery ward, and the private ob-gyns are only responsible for the prenatal care.

Laborists are not pressured to expedite deliveries because they do not have patients waiting to be seen in the office or other obligations. They can allow labor to progress naturally, with less intervention. Cesarean rates are lower—down 25 percent—and vaginal birth after cesarean (VBAC) rates are higher in hospitals that use laborists.

If you plan on a hospital birth, you should ask your doctor whether your hospital employs laborists and what their role is. In most cases, you will not be able to meet a laborist ahead of time. They work in shifts, so you will be assigned the available doctor for that day. As a result, some patients worry they will feel uncomfortable with a doctor they have never met. However, surveys of patients who have used a laborist find a high level of satisfaction with this system.

Working with a Doctor

While prenatal care is standardized across the United States, women's experiences with their doctor depends on the doctor's practice style. Practice patterns vary tremendously from doctor to doctor, from hospital to hospital, and from state to state. If you are interested in a noninterventional birth, you should ask your doctor about his philosophy early in the pregnancy.

Prenatal Care

Your prenatal care with an OB will include a series of office visits every two to four weeks. Believe it or not, an average visit with an OB lasts six minutes. The visits are short because the doctor sees many patients during the day and also balances appointment hours with the time he needs for patients in labor. For example, if a woman is ready to deliver during office hours, the doctor will need to leave patients waiting in the office while he attends the delivery. The delivery can take anywhere from fifteen minutes to a few hours. A doctor may feel pressured to complete the delivery quickly so as to accommodate the women who are waiting to be seen in the office.

Labor

While you are in labor, you may only see your doctor briefly, sometimes not until it is time to deliver. Of course, if there is any concern about the progress of your labor or issues with the baby, the doctor will arrive sooner. The doctor can usually monitor your baby's heart rate remotely on a computer or cell phone from the office or from home. Your nurse and doctor will be in contact many times during labor to discuss its progress. If you are having your first baby, your nurse may even start pushing with you before your doctor comes to the hospital, since some first-time moms have to push for hours. Second and third babies, on the other hand, usually come out within fifteen to twenty minutes. As you get closer to the delivery, the doctor will be notified that it is time to come to "catch the baby."

The Advantage of Having a Doctor at Your Delivery

There are advantages to having a doctor deliver your baby.

- He is trained and prepared for any outcome.
- A doctor has extensive experience. On average, an ob-gyn delivers 8 to 10 babies per month.
- A doctor can deal with any complication that arises.
- A doctor can care for high-risk pregnancies.
- He can perform a cesarean, or use forceps and vacuum.

The Disadvantages of Working with a Doctor

- A doctor is influenced by his training, malpractice fears, and numerous regulations.
- A doctor sees multiple patients and is often rushed.
- A doctor is more likely to intervene in the natural process.
- A doctor usually will only be with you during labor when it is time to deliver.

Working with a Midwife

Midwives are professionals who provide prenatal care, deliver babies, and promote natural birth. They view pregnancy and birth as a normal process, try to avoid unnecessary interventions, and are educated to recognize deviations in patterns of normal labor. Midwives are trained to the same standards as physicians in terms of the labor process. They will monitor the baby's heart rate regularly as well as the mother's vital signs. A midwife can deliver babies in a hospital, a birthing center, or at home. Midwives care only for low-risk women and cannot perform surgery. If a pregnancy develops a complication, a midwife will transfer the patient to a physician.

The midwifery model differs from that of an obstetrician. A prenatal visit with a midwife may take an hour, and many of them take place in the home. Midwives support a woman in making decisions about her body and her birth. They are able to give more one-on-one attention during labor without the distraction of a busy office practice. Midwives will focus not only on the physical changes of pregnancy but also on the emotional and psychological effects on the mother and her family.

The World Health Organization (WHO) suggests that women who are low risk may use the services of a midwife. They define *low risk* as:

- The pregnancy is not complicated by medical conditions of the mother or fetus.
- The labor is spontaneous, not induced.
- The labor remains low risk throughout its course.
- The fetus is head down and between 37 and 43 weeks in gestation.

The Three Types of Midwives

In the United States, there are three types of midwives: certified nurse midwives (CNMs), certified professional midwives (CPMs), and lay midwives, who attend 8 percent of the nation's annual births (32,000 per year). Given that there are about 2 million low-risk pregnancies per year, the number of midwives is clearly insufficient to care for all the patients who may want one. In contrast, in the United Kingdom, midwives attend over 80 percent of all births.

Midwifery students in the United States have several options available for their education and testing. Licensing varies from state to state. Knowing your midwife's credentials will help you understand the skills she has been trained in and the extent of treatment she can provide.

AMCB Certification

Governed by the American College of Nurse-Midwives, American Midwife Certification Board (AMCB)–certified midwives work mainly in hospitals, but also may deliver in birth centers or in the home. ACOG recommends that patients only work with a midwife who is AMCB certified.

CNM (certified nurse midwife): A CNM is a registered nurse (RN) who has completed additional training in midwifery. Most CNM programs require the student to obtain a bachelor of science in nursing (BSN) degree, which can be completed in three or four years. She will then earn a master of science in nursing (MSN) degree that has a concentration in midwifery, or a doctoral degree from an accredited midwifery school. This course of study takes an additional two years. There are thirty-nine accredited CNM programs in the United States. A CNM can work in a hospital, write prescriptions, and carry malpractice insurance. She must pass an exam to be certified and must maintain her certification by completing teaching modules every five years. All fifty states grant licenses to CNMs. There are eleven thousand CNMs practicing in the United States.

CM (certified midwife): A CM has completed a bachelor's degree in a field other than nursing, and receives a MSN or doctoral degree from a midwifery school. Certified midwives are licensed only in New Jersey, Rhode Island, New York, Delaware, and Missouri. They take the same certification exam as a CNM. There are two accredited CM programs in the United States.

NARM Certification

The North American Registry of Midwives (NARM) requires midwives to hold a high school diploma but not a college degree.

CPM (certified professional midwife): CPMs only deliver babies outside of a hospital, usually in the home (75 percent of all home births are attended by CPMs). They cannot write prescriptions and generally do not carry malpractice insurance. There are 2,500 CPMs in the United States.

There are two pathways to becoming a CPM: graduate from a midwifery education program or complete the Portfolio Evaluation Process (PEP). A midwifery education program is a school that offers modules online or in a classroom. The program can be completed in three years and involves working with a preceptor for thirty to forty hours per week as well as taking didactic classes. Candidates must pass an exam administered by the North American Registry of Midwives to be certified, and must be recertified every three years. Ten programs in the United States are currently accredited by the Midwifery Education Accreditation Council (MEAC); numerous other programs are nonaccredited. Students who complete the midwifery education program may receive an associate's or bachelor's degree.

The PEP pathway is an apprentice program in which a student works side by side with a midwife preceptor. She will not be granted a degree but can be certified as a CPM if she passes the NARM exam, observes twenty deliveries, and is the primary birth attendant for ten deliveries.

In twenty-seven states, certified professional midwives can also be licensed, giving them the additional designation of licensed midwife (LM). The licensing process varies tremendously from state to state but involves attending a certain number of deliveries and completing skills testing. If a midwife is licensed by her state, she will be able to carry medications to prevent bleeding, start IVs, give IV antibiotics, and administer oxygen.

In the other twenty-three states, CPMs cannot be licensed and therefore must practice "underground." Unlicensed CPMs find it difficult to receive insurance payments, collaborate with physicians, and maintain relationships with a hospital. Technically, an unlicensed CPM can be prosecuted for practicing medicine without a license. The patchwork of laws regulating CPMs makes it difficult for patients to know the qualifications of their provider.

CPMs are not licensed in Alaska, Connecticut, Georgia, Hawaii, Illinois, Iowa, Kansas, Kentucky, Maine, Maryland, Massachusetts, Michigan, Mississippi, Missouri, Nebraska, Nevada, North Carolina, North Dakota, Ohio, Oklahoma, Pennsylvania, South Dakota, and West Virginia.

Only two states—Florida and Indiana—require that CPMs carry malpractice insurance.

Seven states—California, Delaware, Florida, Indiana, Louisiana, New Jersey, and New York—require CPMs to have an agreement with a physician to whom they can transfer patients in an emergency. In addition, seven states—Arizona, Arkansas, California, Louisiana, New Jersey, New York, and South Carolina—have laws that limit a midwife's scope of practice to low-risk births only (no breech, no VBAC, no twins).

Uncertified Lay Midwives

A lay midwife, also known as a direct entry midwife (DEM), has no formal education, certification, or license. Instead, she learns through apprenticeships with other midwives or self-study. There is no information on how many lay midwives are practicing in the United States. They also practice in many parts of the world where there is limited access to modern medical care.

The Advantages of Having a Midwife

The advantages of having a midwife include:

- A midwife has more time to spend with each patient at prenatal visits.
- Midwives feel comfortable with the normal, noninterventional birth process.
- Each midwife has fewer patients at one time than do doctors, so they can get to know patients intimately.

- A midwife may help you avoid medical interventions, such as epidurals, episiotomy, and cesarean.
- She will allow labor to progress naturally.
- A midwife will be more available to you during labor.
- She offers a more personal experience.
- Midwives provide similar outcomes to those of physicians for low-risk pregnancies and births.
- Midwives are trained in the emotional and social aspects of pregnancy.

Disadvantages of Working with a Midwife

- If you have a complication, you will need to transfer to another provider.
- A midwife can't perform a cesarean.
- Some insurance plans don't cover midwives.
- Midwives attend fewer births during their training than physicians.

Collaboration Between Doctors and Midwives

The collaboration between doctors and CNMs has been well established, as CNMs are highly trained and integrated into the healthcare system. According to ACOG, for a doctor to work with a CPM, she should have completed a minimum of three years in a midwifery education program. ACOG does not recognize CPMs who have gone through the PEP program only, even if they are certified, and discourages its physicians from establishing relationships with these midwives. Doctors are also limited by rules of their malpractice insurance carriers. Most carriers will not insure a doctor if he accepts the care of a patient who has been attempting to deliver at home but has a complication, unless he has had prenatal visits with the patient during the pregnancy. The insurance company doesn't want the doctor to be blamed for a complication that occurred before he assumed care of the patient.

Health Insurance Coverage for a Midwife

CNMs can have contracts with insurance companies and Medicaid in the same way that doctors do. If your CNM is part of your insurance network, her fees will be covered as an in-network provider.

For CPMs, insurance and Medicaid coverage varies by state. If the CPM is practicing in a state-licensed birthing center, her fees will be paid by Medicaid. Coverage for private insurance varies by carrier. Many insurance companies will not automatically cover the fees of a CPM in a home birth, but with persistence, some patients have been able to get coverage.

Freebirthing (Unassisted Childbirth)

Freebirthing is delivering a baby without any assistance. Freebirthers believe that birth is inherently safe and relatively painless as long as the medical community doesn't interfere. They attest that prenatal care is unnecessary and can't fix most problems anyway. These mothers do not want to give birth in a hospital or birth center. They affirm that medical intervention does more harm than good and that no birth is completely risk-free. The risks of intervention outweigh the risk of birth itself.

Of 4 million births per year in the United States, approximately seven thousand are unassisted. A study in 1984 on a religious community in Indiana where women freebirthed showed an infant death rate 2.7 times higher and maternal death rate 97 times higher than the state average. In communities with limited access to CPMs, such as states that do not offer licenses, women may choose to birth alone. Others may lack the money to pay a provider or are following their religious beliefs.

Famous freebirthing advocate Janet Fraser of Australia, who runs the Joyous Birth website, lost a daughter in 2009 during a freebirth as a result of an entangled umbilical cord, which likely could have been managed by a birth attendant with some medical training.

Choosing Your Provider

Who is going to deliver your baby may simply be a practical or logistical decision. Your insurance carrier may dictate who you see, or there may only be one hospital conveniently located near your home. If you already have an established relationship with a gynecologist, this doctor may be the logical choice. However, if there are multiple providers in your area, you can do some research to find the doctor or midwife who is right for you.

The first step is to determine whether your pregnancy is inherently high or low risk. If you do not have any medical problems that could complicate the pregnancy, you have the option of choosing a doctor or a midwife. Having high blood pressure, diabetes, or an autoimmune disease, such as lupus, precludes you from using a midwife. In addition, if you smoke or are significantly obese, you should work with a physician.

If you have decided to work with a doctor, you can find a list of providers in your network from your insurance company, ask a friend for a referral, or research physicians online. If you know the hospital where you want to deliver, you can call the labor and delivery unit and ask one of the nurses for a recommendation. Once you find a few possibilities, you can schedule an appointment to meet with the doctor. It's a good idea to note (on paper, tablet, or smartphone) the questions you would like to ask, so you can be sure you have covered everything:

- Are you a board-certified physician?
- Does the hospital use laborists? If so, what is their role?

- What is your philosophy regarding natural birth?
- Is mine a high-risk pregnancy? (You may already know this based on a preexisting medical condition, but it is good to ask this doctor what he considers to be high risk.)
- What is your training? How many births have you attended? (You want your doctor to be board certified, have completed an accredited residency program, and done at least 100 births.)
- Generally, how do you view childbirth? (If you want a natural birth, you need to make sure your doctor is supportive of this, as some physicians choose not to take care of patients who want a noninterventional birth.)
- What are your philosophies on pain relief? (If you know you want an epidural, you should ask the doctor whether he has criteria for when you can get it. If you are looking for a natural birth, make sure the doctor will entertain such ideas as movement, massage, and relaxation in water.)
- Do you work in a group or solo practice? (If you want to only see one doctor, then a solo practice may be better.)
- Who will cover if you are not available? (No matter what, you cannot guarantee that your doctor won't be on vacation or sick when you are in labor. Do your doctor's backup physicians have a similar philosophy to his?)
- Which hospitals do you work in? (Make sure the hospital is convenient and covered by your insurance.)
- Do you accept my insurance?
- If I want a VBAC, do you and the hospital allow them?
- What is your cesarean rate? (These are not published data, so you must find out from the doctor directly. WHO suggests that the cesarean rate should be around 19 percent. If your doctor's rate is higher than this, and especially if it is higher than the US average of 32 percent, you may want to ask why it is so high or consider another provider.)

- What is your opinion about induction? (Some doctors will strictly adhere to the guidelines that inductions are done only for medical reasons.)
- Do you allow a doula? (Some doctors will not work with doulas [see page 89 for more about doulas]).

After you have conducted your interview, you need to assess how you feel about the doctor.

- Is it easy to ask questions?
- Does the doctor take the time to explain things?
- Will the doctor consider your wishes?
- What is your gut feeling about her—how is her bedside manner?
- Does she have any sanctions against her by the medical board? (For a doctor or CNM, this information is available through the website of your state's medical board. For a CPM, there is no resource to allow you to find out.)

If you have determined that you would prefer to work with a midwife, you need to ask her some questions as well.

- Did you go to midwifery school or were you trained as an apprentice?
- Do you hold a license in midwifery?
- Do you deliver in a hospital, birthing center, or at home?
- Who covers for you if you are out of town or unavailable?
- How many deliveries have you done?
- Are you able to determine whether/when it is necessary to go to a hospital?
- What is your transport rate?
- Is there a doctor at the hospital who is your backup?
- Do you accept my insurance?

Remember that there is always a possibility that your pregnancy will develop a complication—preeclampsia, uncontrolled gestational diabetes, a placenta previa, or if your baby is breech—which would mean that you need to transfer care from a midwife to a doctor.

If You Don't Like Your Provider

the doctor's diary

Women need to be better consumers of their prenatal care and hold their provider—whether OB or midwife—to a high standard. You should select a provider who treats you respectfully, takes time to answer your questions, and communicates with you on a level that you understand. He should value your time by being available at your scheduled appointment. Your doctor or midwife should make decisions with you, not for you, and provide information and guidance by navigating between scientific data, personal experiences, and traditional practices in the field. You may find that even a well-respected expert doesn't have a great bedside manner or that the doctor your friend loves isn't a good fit for you.

Five signs you don't have the right provider:

- He is always late or rushes through your appointment.
- He doesn't return your phone calls.
- He minimizes your concerns.
- He becomes defensive when you question him.
- He is not board certified or board eligible, or has been sanctioned by the medical board.

When you are newly pregnant, especially with your first baby, you may not even know what is important to you for your birth. As the pregnancy progresses and you learn more about your options, you may discover that your provider is not supportive of the direction in which you want to go. You are not doing yourself or your provider any favors by staying with him if your philosophies are inherently different. Some doctors are very frank when discussing their rules. They won't take care of patients who decline routine medical interventions. Some don't offer VBACs. Some won't allow you to go past your due date. If having a natural birth is important to you, you will be better off with a doctor whose views match your own, or who is open-minded about working with your choices. Perhaps there isn't a dramatic difference in your approaches to childbirth, but you may feel that your questions aren't being taken seriously. Keep in mind that every provider is different. The doctor may be perfectly fine for your gynecological care but when it comes to your pregnancy, his philosophy doesn't suit what you need now.

No matter how long, or how briefly, you have been working with your doctor, it is your right to find someone who may be a better fit. If you are not happy with your provider during your prenatal visits, the situation isn't likely to improve during labor. As soon as you realize that you would like to make the switch, you should move forward. Some physicians may not accept new patients during the last month of pregnancy, but many do.

If you are unsure you've found the right person, it may be worthwhile to meet a few different providers. You can get referrals from friends, people you have met in a birthing class, or from a doula. You can interview a new provider and be specific about what wasn't working with the first.

To switch, you can simply ask the new provider to request your records. You don't need to have an uncomfortable confrontation with the original provider, unless there is something you'd like to say directly.

Others Involved in Your Birth

Aside from your doctor or midwife, and depending on where you deliver (hospital, home, birthing center), there will be others involved in your birth.

Nurses

Labor and delivery nurses are registered nurses (RNs) who have completed a bachelor of science in nursing degree. While you do not get to choose your nurse, she will be one of the most important people involved in your delivery. She has likely chosen to work on the labor floor or in the birth center because she loves working with women on this incredibly significant day of their life.

Nurses are employees of the hospital. Not knowing how many women will be in labor each day challenges the hospital to properly staff the labor and delivery unit. Two women in early labor will share one nurse who will go back and forth between the two rooms. Once the delivery is imminent, one nurse will stay with one patient through the birth and recovery period. The second laboring patient will be assigned a new nurse. Also at the change of shift (usually at seven a.m. and seven p.m.), a new nurse will assume your care. As a result, you may have multiple nurses during your labor.

Your nurse records your vital signs every hour during early labor and every thirty minutes in active labor. She closely monitors the fetal heart rate tracing (information from the fetal monitor) and interprets it for the doctor. She will ask you about your pain, and whether you would like medication. She will keep you clean, change your position, and notify your doctor about your progress. Her main goal is to make sure that you and your baby are healthy and safe. When there is downtime, your nurse will be able to get to know you, provide emotional support, and offer advice on how you can achieve the goals of your birth. While she may want to support your birth plan as much as possible, she also must follow the guidelines of the hospital and the orders of your doctor.

Doulas

A doula is a person who is trained to offer continuous emotional and physical support to a woman during labor. She is hired by the mother and is accountable only to her. The word *doula* originates from the Greek word for "woman's servant" and was coined in the 1970s. In addition to being with a woman on her big day, a doula will usually meet with her client at least a few times during the pregnancy for preparation and education. Some patients forgo traditional childbirth classes in lieu of a doula's instruction. A doula may also provide postpartum care.

A doula is a modern-day version of the traditional birth support system, which historically was made up of family and friends who would stay with a laboring woman until the baby was born. Unlike your doctor or nurse, a doula will be with you continuously from the beginning of labor until after the delivery. While many patients expect that their nurses will provide emotional support and physical comfort during labor, that is not always the case, as the nurse needs to care for more than one patient at a time and is responsible for documenting the course of labor, taking vital signs, and administering medications. Although doulas do not offer medical advice or perform any clinical tasks, they can alleviate a woman's fear by explaining what is happening throughout labor, and serve as a liaison between you and your doctor. Doulas usually limit themselves to a few clients who are due to deliver each month so they can ensure that they can attend the births.

A doula can be a vital part of the childbirth team, whether you have a natural delivery, an epidural, or a cesarean. If you need a cesarean, most hospitals permit both your doula and partner to be with you during the surgery. Your doula's role in the operating room is equally important, as she is available to explain what to expect and keep you calm.

Hiring a doula is optional, but if you want to have a natural birth, doing so could be advantageous. In medical studies evaluating over fifteen thousand women from sixteen countries, patients who used doulas were more likely to deliver vaginally and 9 percent less likely to use epidurals. Having a doula decreases the chance of a cesarean by 28 percent. Labors were shorter by forty minutes and the use of

Pitocin decreased by 31 percent. Women's satisfaction with birth also increases when using a doula.[1] Women attest that doulas, who give one-to-one care focused on the emotional aspect of labor, are better than a nurse or family member in providing emotional support. Of course, family members can be helpful, but they are usually not experts in childbirth and are often nervous themselves.

Although a doula is not required to be licensed, many of them are certified through such organizations as the Childbirth and Postpartum Professional Association (CAPPA) or Doulas of North America (DONA). The certification usually includes attending workshops, proof of attending births with another doula, and recommendations from families. In 1994, DONA had 750 certified doulas. By 2012, that number had increased to 6,154.

Only 5 to 10 percent of pregnant women in the United States hire a doula. Many women say they would like to have one but can't afford it or don't know where to find one. Almost half of pregnant women are not familiar with the idea of a doula at all. You can find a doula through a referral from your doctor or a friend or the DONA website, www.dona.org.

Cost of hiring a doula: A doula may charge a few hundred to a few thousand dollars, depending on your location and her experience. However, the total cost of maternity care is $1,000 less when a patient uses the services of a doula because fewer babies are born prematurely or by cesarean.[2]

the doctor's diary

When I began working in private practice in the late 1990s, I had my first encounter with doulas. This was a time when cesarean rates were climbing rapidly, continuous fetal monitoring was the norm, and birth was quite "medicalized." As a result of these trends, many doulas felt that they needed to adamantly stand up for their patients; this, in turn, fostered a climate of distrust between doulas and doctors. Some doulas would question my judgment in front of the patients. I even worked with a doula who made my patient feel terrible about wanting an epidural and walked out when she got it.

As is the case in any profession, not every doula makes the birthing experience better. I have seen doulas who fell asleep during a long labor. I have worked with others who, while advocating for their patient, argue with the medical staff. I have seen doulas who have driven a wedge between a patient and her provider, causing the patient to second-guess their doctor's recommendations. In fact, a study in 2006 showed that 44 percent of women found the relationship between their doula and nurses/doctors to be confrontational and hostile. Some hospitals even banned doulas due to the conflicts.

More often, I have seen numerous cases where a doula has been able to keep a mother focused and relaxed in a way that no one else could. Many doulas massage their clients, speak to them softly, help them change positions, wipe their brow, and encourage them with pushing in the perfect way to help them deliver.

In my experience, the relationship between doulas and doctors has improved dramatically over the last ten years. These days, I am relieved to find out that my patient has hired a doula. I find that my patients who work with doulas are much more relaxed and better educated about the birth process. I wish every patient could have one.

Choosing Where to Have Your Baby

Where you deliver your baby can greatly enhance or diminish your experience. Your provider should respect your right to an informed choice about the place of birth. Most women make their decision based on where their provider works and which location is most convenient. The majority of births take place in a hospital where the woman's doctor or midwife practices, where all medical interventions are available, and where there is a nursing staff in attendance. Some women choose to give birth at home or in a birthing center, and the number of those who do is on the rise: the percentage of out-of-hospital births increased from 1.26 percent of US births in 2011 to 1.36 percent in 2012, nearly doubling the rate from 2004.

Choosing a location is also influenced by where you live and the available services in your area. In some communities, birthing centers don't exist, or there aren't enough midwives to attend home births. Insurance will cover most hospitals. Some birthing centers are also covered, if they are accredited. Of course, having your baby at home is free, other than the cost of your midwife.

Hospitals

More than 98 percent of births in the United States take place in hospitals. Similar rates are seen in the United Kingdom, Germany, Japan, Canada, Australia, and France. The only developed country with a lower rate of hospital birth is the Netherlands at 70 percent.

The majority of hospital deliveries—92 percent—are done by doctors, and 8 percent by CNMs or CMs. Most women choose a hospital without too much consideration because it is the social norm in the developed world and is the most trusted and comfortable choice for many families.

Advantage to hospital birth: In a hospital, you have access to medical interventions that can be lifesaving for you and your baby. A hospital provides ob-gyns who can deliver your baby in just a few minutes by cesarean, anesthesiologists who can make your experience pain-free, and pediatricians who can assist your baby with transitioning to life outside the womb. You can use medications, antibiotics, and blood transfusions at a moment's notice. Most hospitals offer epidurals twenty-four hours a day, though some small hospitals may only have an anesthesiologist on call who will come in from home when needed. A newborn nursery is available in nearly all hospitals, but some will also have a neonatal intensive care unit (NICU) that can provide care to the smallest premature babies or those who are critically ill. If your baby has been identified as having any health issues during prenatal care, such as a birth defect or poor fetal growth, you should confirm that your hospital has the appropriate facilities to care for your newborn.

After an uncomplicated vaginal delivery, women are allowed to stay in the hospital forty-eight hours. After a cesarean, they can stay four days. Many new mothers relish this time in the hospital, where they have assistance with breastfeeding, changing diapers, and learning what postpartum changes are normal, but they are allowed to leave earlier if they feel ready and are recovering without complications.

Downside to hospital birth: The hospital model is ideally designed to manage high-risk pregnancies. Extrapolating that model to include low-risk pregnancies has proven difficult. As a result, technologies and medical interventions are applied equally to all births. Hospitals can feel impersonal and the staff attending to a woman in labor, such as nurses or anesthesiologists working in shifts, is inconsistent. Rooms are anything but private with housekeeping personnel emptying your trash, food service workers taking your postpartum dinner order, and other nurses entering your room to look for supplies. Hospitals foster an air of anxiety for some women, who view them as a sterile and unfamiliar place for the sick and dying. Women hoping for a natural birth require physical and emotional support, patience, and privacy. Hospitals are not always able to provide these intangible necessities.

the doctor's diary

When I began my residency at Los Angeles County Hospital in 1995, the atmosphere of the labor and delivery unit could best be described as controlled chaos. At that time, about thirty babies were delivered every day! I had a plan to keep track of each baby I delivered, but that idea quickly faded since I never even had time to write them down.

The labor and delivery unit was staffed by a team of residents and medical students, with attending physicians available for consultation in an adjacent part of the hospital. A patient would labor in a large room along with three other women. Their families, including spouses/partners, were not at the bedside but in a waiting room nearby. When a woman was ready to deliver, the nurse would call a resident to the room.

The mother would be disconnected from her fetal monitors and her bed would be pushed down the hall to the operating room (OR). In the cold OR, she would be transferred from her labor bed to a narrow table. Her legs were placed into stirrups and she would begin pushing with an intern or medical student standing by. A nurse and pediatric team were also available. As a more senior resident, I would run from room to room when my assistance was needed. After each baby was born, the new mother would be moved back to the labor bed, her baby placed in a bassinet, and she would be wheeled to a recovery area. At this point, her husband and family could meet the baby. The operating suite had nine ORs, and sometimes deliveries would be going on in all of them at once. From the sinks in the hallway where we washed our hands, I could hear mothers shouting and groaning as they pushed, interns and nurses coaching, and newborn babies crying.

Thankfully, these high-volume, impersonal delivery units are a thing of the past. Now hospitals strive to make their rooms more comfortable and inviting. Many labor and delivery units offer private rooms, flat-screen TVs, hardwood floors, and Jacuzzi tubs. Women labor, deliver, and recover in the same room. Families are allowed to visit at any time of day. These days, partners stay throughout the process and the mother and baby are rarely separated. In case of an emergency, operating rooms are located on the same floor. In addition, a nursery or NICU is available to help with care of the newborns.

A labor and delivery unit is unique in that a beautiful delivery can take place in one room while, next door, a woman can be grieving a terrible loss. An unprepared teenager is in a room next to a forty-five-year-old woman who has been trying to get pregnant for ten years. It is a place where new families are created.

⊰⊱ LILY'S STORY ⊰⊱

My boyfriend and I were expecting our first baby and were bombarded with questions from friends and family about what kind of birth we wanted. I have been a yoga instructor in Los Angeles for seven years. I'm surrounded every day by fit, health-conscious women. Some of them have taken my class right up until delivery of their own babies. They would often talk about their plans for having a natural birth. A few even had their babies at home, and gushed about the wonderful experience. They spoke of the freedom to move around, the support of their midwives, and the peacefulness of the situation. These natural birthing moms assured me that labor would be a breeze for me since I was so fit.

I didn't have the heart to tell them that I wanted no part of an unmedicated birth. I knew having a Pap smear was uncomfortable for me and I couldn't envision delivering a baby without drugs. I believed that sometimes it's okay to ask for help. That help may come in the form of an epidural in a long labor or letting your baby be taken care of in a nursery for a few hours so you can get some sleep. For me, the prize was a healthy baby. I didn't need another medal for doing it without medication. ⟨⟨

Natural Birth in the Hospital

Without a doubt, a hospital is the safest place for a woman to give birth who has high blood pressure, preterm labor, or a breech baby. But if you do not have any issues that would demand high-risk care, you should find out about your hospital's policies regarding the routine use of IVs, fetal monitoring, movement during labor, and delivery positions. If your hospital is flexible, you can easily have a natural birth with the confidence that any emergency can be easily handled.

⟨⟨ OLIVIA'S STORY ⟩⟩

Olivia, a 35-year-old mom of two, chose to have a natural birth experience in a hospital. Her attitude and preparation were key to her success. She didn't approach labor as a terrifying ordeal but, rather, as an amazing feat she knew her body was capable of. She was influenced by the story of her own birth in which her mother described the experience as gratifying and beautiful. She prepared for each of her labors with the help of her doula. A chiropractor who specializes in pregnancy also gave Olivia deep tissue massages during the last few months of pregnancy to relax her pelvic muscles, which Olivia recalls as being painful but effective in keeping her flexible. She felt most comfortable giving birth in a hospital in case things didn't go as planned. She wasn't against medication on principle—she just preferred to try the natural way, anticipating that it would be bearable. Thanks to her preparation, physical fitness, and lack of fear, it was.

"As I was going through labor, it felt like every contraction prepared me to embrace the next one," she says. "There was never a moment where I said, 'Now I want medication.' It was almost like a bonding experience—I was aware of my baby at every moment and did not want to let drugs mute that feeling." 🍃

Birthing Centers

A birthing center offers a comfortable, relaxed environment for labor, delivery, and postpartum care. It can be freestanding or attached to a hospital. Birthing centers are designed to accommodate women with low-risk pregnancies receiving care from a midwife. They are stocked with basic emergency supplies such as IVs, oxygen, and medication to control bleeding. They are committed to keeping families together during this exciting event. A birthing center is the perfect alternative for women who want to give birth in an intimate environment but don't feel comfortable or do not want to have their baby in their own home.

Women who deliver in a birthing center will typically stay for a few hours after the birth and then go home to continue their recovery. The center is not designed to have women stay for more than a day after the delivery. The quick discharge from a birthing center may be challenging for a new mom, who needs some time to rest and transition to her new role.

There are 313 birthing centers in United States—an increase of 57 percent since 2010. About sixteen thousand babies per year are born in birthing centers—about 0.4 percent of US births. Twenty percent of these centers are owned by or affiliated with hospitals. The others are freestanding facilities.

The Commission for the Accreditation of Birth Centers (CABC) certifies the centers. However, only one third of centers in the United States have been certified. The majority of birth centers operate without this accreditation because they do not meet the commission's criteria for safety or they are unable to obtain a transfer agreement with a hospital for emergencies. Without an agreement in place, the midwife would be left to call 911 or to take the patient to the nearest emergency room.

Accredited centers only allow delivery for low-risk patients. They do not allow breech births, twin deliveries, or labor induction. Some centers can accommodate VBACs if certain criteria are met. Monitoring of the fetal heart rate is done intermittently— every thirty minutes during active labor and every five to fifteen minutes during the pushing phase. Pain relief options at a birth center include water immersion in a tub, movement, massage, and nitrous oxide.

The location of a birth center is important in determining its safety. Nearly 80 percent of the accredited centers are within a thirty-minute drive of a hospital. Of course, preventing emergencies from happening in the first place should be done by carefully screening potential clients, having a well-rehearsed emergency drill, initiating treatment during transport, and having a receiving hospital available. If a birth center is accredited, you can feel confident that these things are part of the protocol. The chance of a baby's dying during childbirth in an accredited center is 0.8 per 1,000.

The actual, "rack rate" cost of delivering in a birth center is about one third the cost of delivering in a hospital. A hospital birth with no complications (not including newborn charges) costs $10,000 and a birth center costs $3,000. Depending on the terms of your insurance, the out-of-pocket costs for you may or may not be lower. With the Affordable Care Act, Medicaid is now required to cover the fees at state-licensed freestanding birthing centers. Many private insurers are following suit.

A 2013 study of accredited birthing centers showed the following outcomes: [3]

- 94% of patients had a vaginal birth.
- 16% of patients were transferred to a hospital.
- 98% of transfers were for non-emergent reasons.

Advantage: Birth centers strive to create a comfortable, homelike environment. They offer privacy, and less chance of needing a cesarean. Some medical interventions are available.

Disadvantages: In a birthing center, you will be discharged within a few hours of delivery. They are only equipped to handle normal labors, so if you have a complication, you would need to be transferred.

❧ TRACEY'S STORY ❧

I chose to have my baby in a birthing center and it was the best decision I have ever made. I have always been nervous about being in a hospital. After doing lots of research, I thought that a birthing center might be a better option for me. My pregnancy was great, no problems at all. The midwives at the center explained how the center works, what credentials they have, and what situations would require them to transfer me to the hospital. We found out that my insurance wouldn't cover the birthing center because I didn't have any out-of-network benefits. The total cost was $6,500 for my prenatal care and delivery. The money was definitely an issue, but my husband and I decided it was worth it.

A week after my due date, during lunch, I felt my first contractions. They were mild but it was clear that something different was happening. I went home, and within a few hours, I was breaking a sweat with each contraction. I called my midwife, and she told me to head to the birthing center.

The room at the center looked just like a bedroom. The lights were dim, soft music was playing, and the bed was made with lots of fluffy pillows. My midwife turned on the bubbles in the in-room Jacuzzi. I spent the next few hours in and out of the tub, walking around the room, and lying on the bed when it felt good. The midwife would check my baby's heartbeat on and off, and he always sounded strong.

The pain got really crazy at one point. I told my midwife I didn't know how much longer I could go like this. But she assured me that it was normal, and that it was almost over. For a brief moment, I did think about having my husband drive me to the hospital, but I found a new energy when I felt like I needed to go to the bathroom. My midwife said this was probably the baby's head, and that I should bear down with the contraction. It actually felt really good to push and distracted me from the pain. She told me to sway from side to side as I pushed. I felt like I was wiggling my son out. It seemed like forever, and it actually was almost two hours that I pushed.

My son was born after sixteen hours of labor, weighing 8 pounds. I held him on my chest and my midwife showed me how to help him latch on. We stayed in the birthing center for six hours and then went home. I was a little nervous being at home alone with him, but my midwife assured me I was doing great. She was just a phone call away.

I loved my birthing experience. Compared to the stories of my friends who had hospital births, it seemed so peaceful. My only wish is that we could have stayed there a little longer! 🌿

Home Birth

One percent of births in the United States (36,000 per year) happen at home. Of these, 75 percent are planned home births and 25 percent happen accidently because the woman didn't make it to the hospital in time. While the number of women choosing home birth is still low, it has increased by 70 percent from 2004 to 2015. In Alaska, Idaho, Oregon, Pennsylvania, Washington, and Wyoming, more than 3 percent of births occur in the home. Most home births (75 percent) are attended by CPMs and lay midwives.

Why Women Choose Home Birth

Educated, middle- to upper-income, Caucasian women are most likely to choose a home birth. Many have become skeptical of modern medicine and want to rely on their intuition for childbirth. For others, being in a hospital is uncomfortable and unfamiliar. In light of the horror stories of other women's hospital births discussed around the water cooler at work or on the Internet, there is no doubt that women want an alternative. When hospitals no longer offer women such options as VBAC or the vaginal delivery of twins and breech babies, some patients, particularly those who don't have access to a birth center or whose insurance won't cover the costs, may feel that their only choice is home birth. Women wanting a natural birth are skeptical that hospitals can provide a peaceful, unmedicated experience.

Birthing at home helps women feel they can retain control over their body. Twenty percent of women who have given birth in a hospital say they would consider a home birth for their next pregnancy because of a negative experience the first time. This sentiment especially rings true for patients who had a cesarean. If a woman feels that her first birth was fraught with tension and discord because of the inflexible attitudes of hospital staff and/or hospital policies that led to a cesarean, she may feel that the only way to avoid a second one is to give birth at home.

In theory, home birth sounds like a wonderful prospect. The people surrounding you are invited family and friends, as well as your doula and midwife with whom you have bonded over the last nine months. If your home is a special, comfortable, nourishing space for you, a home birth may be in order.

Advantages: comfort, more freedom, no time restrictions, privacy, low cost, continuous one-on-one care, less chance of interventions (such as episiotomy, cesarean, epidural).

Disadvantages: must be transported to a hospital for an emergency, minimal medical equipment or medications readily available, the chance of a baby dying during labor or having a serious complication is higher.

Research on Home Births

Most studies on home birth were conducted in European countries where midwifery training and the integration of midwives into the health-care system are different than they are in the United States. Research on the relative risks of home birth versus hospital birth is difficult to conduct because women cannot be forced to have one type of birth or another. Birth statistics alone don't account for the women who attempted to deliver at home but were transferred to the hospital. In addition, many studies don't distinguish between planned and unintended home births. It is important to remember that, in the hospital, there may also be risks that go along with various interventions that are not reflected directly in the neonatal and maternal mortality rates.

Two large studies in Europe show home and hospital birth to be equally safe for mothers who have given birth before. For first-time mothers, the risk of the baby having a severe complication was higher at home, yet still well less than 1 percent.[4] The cesarean rate in the hospital was four to eight times higher than at home, which indicates that the risk of overintervention in a hospital may outweigh the risk of underintervention at home.[5]

Studies conducted in the United States, however, consistently show that babies born at home have a two to four times higher chance of dying than those born in a hospital. A study conducted by the Midwives Alliance of North America (MANA) in the *Journal of Midwifery* in 2014 showed that the risk of a baby born at home dying during labor or during the first month of life was 2.06 per thousand,[6] whereas the risk in a hospital is 0.4 per thousand.[7] One of the reasons that home birth in the United States is more dangerous is that many patients who give birth at home are not truly low-risk. When the high-risk patients are removed from the statistics, the risk decreases to 1.61 per thousand. Similarly, in a review of birth data from Oregon (which is the only state to publish information on home births), 75 percent of the neonatal deaths that occurred at home were to women with high-risk pregnancies, such as twins, breech, and VBAC.[8]

Who Is a Candidate for a Home Birth?

According to ACOG and AAP (American Academy of Pediatrics), as well as organizations in numerous European countries, you are a candidate for home birth if:

- You are between 37 and 42 weeks.
- You have no preexisting diseases or pregnancy complications.

- You have never had a cesarean.
- You are having one baby.
- Your baby is head down.
- Your baby has not passed meconium.
- Your water has not been broken for more than 24 hours.

In the United States, 9 to 30 percent of the home births that occur do not fit these criteria. One in 135 home births is of a breech baby. In 1 in 22, a woman is attempting a VBAC. One in 156 women giving birth at home is carrying twins.

Cost

The cost of having your baby at home is only the fee you pay to your midwife. Most insurance companies and Medicaid do not cover CPMs or lay midwives. Some CNMs have contracts with insurance companies, but most do not. The price for prenatal care and delivery at home ranges from $1,500 to $8,000. If your insurance policy offers out-of-network coverage, the company may consider the midwife an out-of-network provider and, if you submit a claim, reimburse a portion of the fee.

Transfer Rates for Home Births

Many women who set out to have a home birth ultimately end up delivering in a hospital. First-time moms attempting to give birth at home transfer to a hospital 30 to 40 percent of the time. If you've had a baby before, the transfer rate is 5 to 10 percent.[9] Transfers happen because of slow progress in labor, fetal heart rate abnormalities, the need for pain relief, high blood pressure, bleeding after the delivery, or issues with the newborn. The vast majority of transfers are not for emergencies.

The relationship between home birth midwives and doctors/ hospitals is generally strained. In nearly half of US states, CPMs are practicing without a license and are unsupported by the general medical system. Many doctors and nurses feel strongly that home birth is dangerous. The stigma of a "failed home birth" causes many women and their midwives to stay home as long as possible. When a woman transfers, the hospital staff may make her feel that her attempt at home birth was a poor decision. The Emergency Medical Treatment and Active Labor Act (1986) ensures emergency care to anyone in labor regardless of her birth preferences or ability to pay.

Home Birth in Other Countries

In the United Kingdom, the Netherlands, Australia, and Canada, clear guidelines designate who is a candidate for home birth.

In the United Kingdom, a woman who wants a home birth will also register at a hospital and be assigned a doctor. That way, if she needs to transfer, there is an easy path to emergency care. The Netherlands boasts the highest home birth rate in the developed world: 30 percent of babies are born at home with the supervision of a midwife. Here, midwife training is rigorous, competitive, and uniform. Midwives have specific relationships with doctors and are fully integrated into the health-care system.

Preparing for a Home Birth

the doctor's diary

As a mother, you must be realistic about your pregnancy. Just because you really want to have a home birth doesn't mean that you can ignore obvious facts. If your baby is breech, if you have twins or high blood pressure, you should deliver in the safest possible environment with the most skilled practitioner. That environment is not going to be your home.

And just because a midwife agrees to do a home birth doesn't make it safe. The best midwife is someone who can recognize when it is time to transfer to the hospital.

If you are having a home birth, your plan must include a hospital option as well. Research the nearest hospital and find out how long it takes you to get there. Confirm that there will be a doctor available and willing to care for you in an emergency.

You need to decide ahead of time what part of the house you want to deliver in. Most women choose their bedroom, but some may prefer a comfortable den or living room. Once you have decided on the location, you can start to de-clutter this area and create the space you envision. You should also think about who will be present during the delivery. If you have other children, you should consider their maturity and how prepared they are for the event. Watching birth videos may be a great way to introduce the concepts. You should plan to have a friend or family member in attendance to care for your children in case they become uncomfortable during your labor or you need to be transferred to the hospital.

Your midwife will likely give you a list of supplies to have on hand. These include gauze pads, lubricant, and a plastic mattress protector or shower curtain. Most supplies can be ordered online as a "Home Birth Kit," which contains almost everything you will need. Some midwives request you have a clean cookie sheet or tray on which she can arrange her instruments so that she can easily carry them to different areas of the house, in case you decide to deliver in a different room. You will also provide a large bowl for the placenta.

When you are in labor at home, especially during transition, it is common to think that you can't do it. You may even tell your midwife that you want to go to the hospital to get an epidural. Many women say this, but only some really mean it. Since you are close to delivery, you are better served staying where you are.

⇥ KATHERINE'S STORY ⇤

When I was younger, I had no idea that you could have a baby at home. Childbirth sounded scary and very painful. And I knew you could die. During my twenties, I began meeting people who had a more holistic, healthy approach toward life and

I found a loving, nurturing community of friends. I started to think of life as cause and effect. I ate better and indulged less. I knew that if I ever became pregnant, I would care for my body and baby in the same way. Some of my friends had wonderful home birth experiences, so when we decided to start a family, I knew this was the route I wanted to take.

At first, I saw both a doctor and a midwife. My midwife made me feel comfortable and was experienced in water birth so I stopped seeing the physician at twenty weeks. I hired a doula and took hypnobirthing classes, as well as traditional childbirth classes. All of these were essential to the success of my home birth. My midwife monitored me throughout the pregnancy and concluded that I was a good candidate to birth at home.

My water broke at three a.m. two weeks before my due date. I called my midwife. Because I wasn't having strong contractions, she suggested that I try to go back to sleep. I napped on and off until nine a.m. Then I had breakfast and walked around. My contractions became more regular and my midwife arrived at four p.m. She checked my vitals and the baby's heartbeat but did not do a vaginal exam. Active labor really kicked in at ten p.m. and I got in and out of the tub. Originally I wanted to do a water birth, but when the time came, I didn't feel comfortable pushing in the tub, so I lay on my bed on my side. It seemed to be the only position that felt good. My midwife suggested I try the birthing stool, so I moved there. My son was born a few minutes later.

I never felt scared or the need to go to the hospital. I was calm and prepared. I felt pain and it was incredibly difficult at times. But my midwife checked my son's heartbeat, which was always very strong. Knowing that he was okay gave me the strength and confidence to keep going. Feeling supported by my midwife and doula made all the difference. Having the peaceful environment was my favorite part of my home birth, especially for that first magical hour with my son.

Home Versus Hospital: The War of Words

No topic in the field of obstetrics is more polarizing than the debate about home birth. Home birth and hospital birth advocates go head to head regularly about which venue is safer and better for women and their babies. A war of words is being waged on blogs, Twitter, through academic papers, and the media about where a woman should have her baby. The controversy is based on the potential risks of injuries to newborns born at home versus the risks of medical interventions in the hospital. In 2015, an international group of scientists studying home births advised obstetricians that they have the professional responsibility to explain the increased risk of home birth to their patients and to recommend against it.[10] Ultimately, birth safety is not just about numbers, but doing what is best for a mother and her unborn child. Each side can manipulate statistics to advance its opinion.

the doctor's diary

I understand why women choose to deliver in the comfort of their own home. I find many of my physician colleagues recommend interventions just because it's the way it has always been done and are inflexible when it comes to changing protocols. Even things proven to be medically sound—such as having skin-to-skin contact immediately after delivery, encouraging babies to room in with their mothers, keeping the lights dim and distractions to a minimum during labor—are not being implemented across the country. We tell women throughout pregnancy not to use unnecessary medications, not to lie on their back, and to stay active. Then, as soon as they are in labor in the hospital, we give them medicine, put them in bed, and keep them on their back for hours. These contradictions have made some mothers feel that they don't have any other choice than to deliver at home so as to have the birth they want.

When obstetricians compare outcomes for different birth locations, they focus on one thing—how many babies die as a result of being born at home. Home birth advocates, on the other hand, look at the risks of complications from medical interventions and the overall birth experience. Do the risks of overintervention outweigh those of underintervention? How does the consequence of a complication from an unnecessary cesarean stack up against a complication from a birth that permanently injures a child? There is no absolute answer to these questions, and I know the debate will rage on.

I believe that home birth is a legitimate option for women who are truly low risk and well informed, especially if they have given birth before, if they choose a well-qualified midwife, and if they live near a hospital. Having more women attempting to give birth at home will force the obstetrical community to create systems that integrate home birth into mainstream health care.

With standardized training and certification of home birth midwives, the process could be even safer. In addition, I hope the movement toward home birth will encourage doctors to use fewer interventions when possible, so that patients will feel that they can have the birth they envision in the hospital setting as well.

Choosing a Childbirth Style

Numerous birthing techniques offer guidance to women seeking a natural experience. Studies have shown that women who take childbirth preparation classes are less likely to need pain medication, have shorter labors, and are more satisfied with their births. However, there are no data to prove that one method is more effective than the next.

The Alexander Technique

Frederick Alexander pioneered this technique in the early 1900s. It consists of a series of exercises and breathing patterns that relieve muscle tension to improve balance, flexibility, and coordination. It has been used to treat back pain, reduce stress, and improve posture as well as enhance the effectiveness of pushing during labor. Women are taught how to cope with labor pains rather than eliminate them, by consciously releasing involuntary muscle tension. Classes are taught by certified instructors, last thirty to forty-five minutes, and span twelve weeks.

The Bradley Method

The Bradley method is a childbirth education program developed in 1947 by Dr. Robert Bradley of Denver, Colorado. Bradley grew up on a farm watching the birthing patterns of animals. He noted their breathing and the "nests" they created for birth. From these observations, he concluded that birth needs to occur in a quiet, safe place.

Dr. Bradley was one of the first physicians to suggest that a husband needs to be at his wife's side during labor. Of course, "husband" doesn't have to be a husband—it is anyone who can help, other than a doctor. This support person is trained to respond to the mother's emotional and physical needs.

The Bradley method encourages a mother to trust her body and focus on a healthy diet and exercise during pregnancy. She must practice relaxation techniques daily with cues from her partner's voice and touch. In labor, she has six goals: abdominal breathing, quiet, darkness, physical comfort, eyes closed, and deep relaxation.

Some women have found this method to be rigid, leading them to feel guilty if they abandon it and use pain medication.

The Bradley website claims that 86 percent of its patients have an unmedicated, spontaneous birth, although there are no studies to support this statement. Bradley instructors are certified in these techniques and offer twelve-week birthing classes to women and their partners.

Hospital Birthing Classes

Classes offered by the hospital where you plan to deliver include a hospital tour, cover the basics of medical interventions, and explain pain medication options. Most hospital birthing classes do not teach specific techniques to achieve a natural birth but focus instead on explaining what happens in labor and the postpartum.

Hypnobirthing

Hypnosis has been around for centuries but only since the 1990s have women used this technique to alleviate the pain of childbirth. This method focuses on relaxation via self-hypnosis to control the degree of pain and release fears about childbirth. It also teaches mothers how to use music, visualization, or mantras for relaxation. Hypnobirthing classes usually consist of five classes of two to three hours each. Free podcasts and audio downloads are also available to facilitate practice at home.

Studies show that hypnosis reduces the use of epidurals by 50 percent. It may also lower cesarean rates, shorten labor, and provide more satisfaction with the birth.

The Lamaze Method

In the 1940s, Dr. Fernand Lamaze of France developed a childbirth method that uses the mind (psyche) to distract a woman from the pain through breathing and relaxation techniques.

There are six care practices that form the core of the Lamaze method:

1. Encourage natural initiation of labor (no induction; no Pitocin).
2. Employ movement, massage, hot and cold packs, and breathing techniques.
3. Have a support person.
4. Avoid intervention that isn't medically necessary.
5. Avoid birthing on your back and follow your body's urges to push.
6. Keep mom and baby together.

Lamaze Breathing

In the past, the Lamaze technique taught the "hee-hee-hee" breathing that is often depicted in movies. The technique has been modified to "conscious breathing," which is a slow inhale for five seconds with an exhale for five seconds. By focusing on the breath at all times, a mother is distracted from her pain. There are no rules on how many breaths per minute to take or whether to breathe through the nose or mouth; do whatever feels good.

The Leboyer Method

Dr. Frederick Leboyer of France wrote *Birth Without Violence* in 1975. His teachings are not childbirth preparation per se but instead focus on minimizing trauma to the newborn. He discouraged doctors from slapping the baby or hanging it upside down, which, at that time, were common practices to encourage babies to cry and breathe. He believed that a baby should be born in a stress-free environment. The birthing room should be warm and dim so there is less shock to the eyes. Quiet music should be played and visitors should whisper. The baby should be handled gently as the head is allowed to deliver on its own without the doctor's pulling it. The baby should be placed in a warm bath or on the mother's abdomen and massaged to ease crying.

Preparing a Birth Plan

A birth plan is a written document that outlines your preferences during labor. It should reflect how your doctor and hospital staff can help you have a positive birth experience. Some women know exactly what they want from the beginning of pregnancy, while others don't know what the choices are. Think of researching and writing a birth plan as an opportunity to discover which options you want or would prefer to avoid. Birth plans separate women into two general groups: those who want minimal intervention and those who want everything the hospital has to offer. If you know that you prefer to be induced, have a scheduled cesarean, or want an epidural the moment you arrive at the hospital, your birth plan will be quite simple.

If you are interested in having minimal medical interventions, you should find out your doctor's philosophy on this early in pregnancy. Don't wait to have the discussion at thirty-six weeks when you hand your doctor a list of things you want to avoid, only to find out that your doctor or hospital cannot accommodate your wishes. If you are developing a birth plan to "protect" yourself from your provider or from the hospital, you should consider finding a new provider or changing the location for your delivery.

Birth plans should be personal. Many patients download a generic birth plan from the Internet and proceed to check a series of boxes about topics that they may not even understand. If you are writing a birth plan, you must understand what you want and why—not just because your friend told you not to get an epidural or your sister suggested that you should deliver standing up. Think about what works for you.

Some choices in these plans are obvious. No one opts for a large episiotomy or chooses to be separated from her baby after birth. If you haven't given birth before, you may not know that many of the options are linked together as a group and aren't independent. For example, if you have an epidural, you can't decline an IV or continuous fetal monitoring and you must stay in bed (because you are connected to the monitor by a 4-foot cord). Many checklist-style plans include such practices as enemas and pubic hair shaving, which are outdated. These generic plans are more useful as a tool to familiarize yourself with common concepts during labor so that you can further research and discuss with your doctor.

Value of a Birth Plan

Having a thoughtfully designed birth plan allows you to learn about the birth process and identify any questions you may have. By doing this, you will feel more confident about what to expect during labor and delivery. It is always better to explore your options during pregnancy, because once you are in labor, things can happen quickly and you may not have time for detailed discussions.

Another important role of the birth plan in modern obstetrics is that it constantly reiterates to us physicians that many patients prefer childbirth to take its natural course. Most birth plans contain such requests as being able to eat and drink during labor, having freedom of movement and birthing positions, allowing labor to progress on its own, and avoiding a cesarean unless medically necessary. In fact, medical research supports all of these requests. Yet, they are still thought of as exceptions to the rule by many obstetricians. With more patients using birth plans, the philosophy of doctors may change so that these special requests ultimately become the norm.

the doctor's diary

Many providers joke that the greater the detail in a birth plan, the higher chance of a cesarean. However, I find that a woman with a birth plan is the ideal patient to work with because she has done her research and has taken the time to think about what is important to her.

You need to speak from the heart in your birth plan—what is really important about your birth? What would an ideal birth look like? Less important is to control every detail of the process. A series of boxes to check, such as "I don't want an IV" or "I only want a cesarean if it is necessary," doesn't help your doctor understand you.

If your labor takes an unexpected turn, what you have written in your plan will not stop your doctor from offering or proceeding with an appropriate intervention. That being said, you may want to include instructions in your birth plan stating that you want to be informed about any changes, why any particular intervention is recommended, and not have interventions without your consent.

Having a great birth experience is not about your doctor's being able to meet a litany of requests. Instead, your plan should reflect how you want to receive information (do you want all the details or just the big picture), what giving consent means to you, what makes you feel safe and respected, what kind of contact and touch is helpful. Even if you don't want pain medication and end up with an epidural, you can feel satisfied with your birth if these other important aspects are met.

Birth plans also need to be fluid. After twenty-four hours of labor, you may feel differently about certain interventions than you did at the twelve-hour mark. Don't use your birth plan as a bar that you've set for yourself. Give yourself permission to change course.

Common Aspects of a Checklist-Style Birth Plan

A generic birth plan can lay out options, but how do you know what is the best choice for you? While the cookie-cutter approach isn't generally helpful, these questions can be a springboard for further research, soul-searching, and discussion with your doctor or midwife. Each of these topics and their pros and cons are discussed in detail later in this book.

During Labor

- Do you want to be able to eat and drink?
- Do you want to be able to move around?
- Do you want the baby to be monitored continuously or intermittently?
- Do you want to wear your own clothes or a hospital gown?
- Who will be at your delivery? Partner/friend/mother/doula/others?
- What are your plans for pain relief?
- Would you like to labor in a tub or shower if one is available?

During Pushing

- Do you prefer an episiotomy or to tear naturally?
- Do you want the staff to coach you while you are pushing or be allowed to follow your instincts?
- Would you prefer a certain position during pushing?

After Delivery

- Do you want your baby to be placed on your skin after birth?
- Do you want the cord to be cut immediately or wait until it stops pulsating?
- Do you want the baby to have the vitamin K shot and antibiotic eye ointment?
- Do you plan to breastfeed?

The very first time I was handed a birth plan, it was four pages long, had multiple colors and font types, and was laminated. The plan outlined every possible detail about the experience along with mini-biographies of each person who would be attending the birth and what their role would be: "Adina—a childhood friend—will be taking still photos. Belinda—my sister-in-law—will be shooting video." My immediate impression was that my patient wanted to control the birth and didn't trust me to do my job. It was as if I were orchestrating an opposing plan for her to have a terrible birth experience.

I did everything I could to help my patient achieve her goals of an unmedicated birth. But ultimately, she was handed a labor that lasted for thirty-six hours, and she decided to have an epidural. She was exhausted, could no longer manage her pain, and hoped the epidural would aid in her delivery. Her support group went home to sleep and she delivered her baby vaginally, legs in stirrups, with an IV, with only her husband present.

Her birth was nothing like what she had envisioned. She had a carefully constructed birth plan, but was willing and able to adjust as her situation changed. Her experience wasn't any less wonderful—simply different than she had anticipated. Ultimately, she was elated to have her baby and completely forgot about all the things that she thought would have been important. She felt good about her choices although they didn't match what she put down in her original plan.

How to Compose a Birth Plan

- Ask your doctor whether she has any "rules" about your labor—does she require you to be continuously monitored? Can you walk around? Can you eat? Do you have to have an IV? If your doctor has specific rules, you can inquire about her reasoning behind them and decide whether they are reasonable for you.
- Does your hospital have specific protocols, such as how many people can be in the room or what happens to your baby immediately after the birth? If there are policies that don't align with your vision, you can ask whether they are flexible or consider finding another venue.

- Think about what you fear about labor. Are you afraid that something bad may happen to your baby? Are you more fearful that a medical intervention could cause a complication? Are you afraid you will not be able to tolerate the pain? Are you nervous about losing control of the decision-making process? Describing your specific fears will help your doctor and health-care team alleviate them.
- If you knew that you and your baby would be healthy and safe at the end, what would your perfect birth look like?
- If an intervention becomes urgently necessary during labor, how can you find out about its risks, benefits, and alternatives? Can your doctor promise to have a brief conversation with you or your partner? Let your doctor know how you can best feel part of the decision.
- As you develop your plan, discuss your philosophy with your doctor and listen equally to hers. Make sure that she knows that you are flexible and willing to accept her recommendations just as she can be flexible with you.

Your birth plan may be as simple as:

We would like to have a natural birth with minimal medical interventions. If an intervention is suggested, we would like to know how it will help, what are its risks, and whether there are any alternatives.

By carefully choosing your provider, selecting the location of your birth, and spending time thinking about what you feel you will need during labor and delivery, you will go a long way toward having the birth experience you desire.

IS THIS TEST OR INTERVENTION NECESSARY?

S CREENING TESTS ARE PERFORMED IN ALL FIELDS OF MEDICINE TO identify diseases before symptoms develop. Common screening tests include mammograms, colonoscopies, and blood tests for cholesterol. During the course of pregnancy, your doctor will suggest a number of screening tests to monitor your health and that of your baby. If you have any medical conditions or if any diseases run in your family, you may require additional diagnostic testing.

Tests you must have include:

Blood type	Rubella
Complete blood count (CBC)	Urine culture
Hepatitis B	Diabetes screening
Human immunodeficiency virus (HIV)	Group B streptococcus (GBS) screening
Rapid plasma reagin (RPR)	

Tests that are optional for women with low-risk pregnancies include:

Human papillomavirus (HPV)	Ultrasound
Pap smear	Cervical exams
Maternal genetic tests	Antepartum testing
Fetal genetic tests	Kick counts

Common Prenatal Tests

Your doctor or midwife will perform these screening tests at each prenatal visit:

Blood pressure: To screen for preeclampsia
Fundal height: To monitor the fetal growth
Urine test for protein: To screen for preeclampsia
Fetal heart rate: By Doppler

Other Screening Tests

The following screening tests identify conditions that could affect your baby.

Blood Type

A mother's blood type is checked, via a blood test, to determine whether she is at risk for a serious condition called isoimmunization, in which she produces antibodies that can attack her own baby, leading to anemia, swelling, and even fetal death. Only women who have a blood type that is Rh negative are at risk.

Our blood cells have proteins on the surface that determine our blood type. Some of these proteins establish our blood group of A, B, or O. Another important protein is called the Rh factor. If you have the Rh factor on your blood cells, you are Rh positive. If you don't

====== **LISTENING TO YOUR BABY'S HEARTBEAT** ======

Listening to your baby's heartbeat allows your doctor to confirm that your baby is alive and that its heart rate is normal. It doesn't tell us how "strong" the heartbeat is or how healthy the baby is. Conventional stethoscopes cannot detect the fetal heartbeat because the heart is deep inside the mother's body, protected by the thick muscular wall of the uterus and cushioned by amniotic fluid. Fetoscopes, also known as Pinard horns, were invented in the 1800s to hear the baby's heartbeat and are still commonly used in Europe. This instrument, which is 8 inches long, hollow, and shaped like a trumpet, can be used after twenty weeks.

In the United States, a Doppler—a handheld ultrasound transducer that utilizes the "Doppler effect" to provide audible simulation of the heartbeat—can detect the fetal heartbeat after twelve weeks.

have this protein, you are Rh negative. Seven percent of Americans are Rh negative. A baby inherits its blood type from its mother or its father. If a mother is Rh negative, and her fetus is Rh positive because it inherited the Rh factor from its father, the mother's immune system recognizes this protein as "foreign" and produces antibodies to attack it.

Isoimmunization only happens when a mother's blood mixes with her baby's. Because mother and baby have two separate circulations, mixing occurs infrequently during pregnancy. At the time of delivery, maternal and fetal blood are more likely to mix, so the antibodies form after the baby is born. The mother carries these antibodies for the rest of her life. If she becomes pregnant again with an Rh-positive baby, those antibodies will immediately attack the second baby.

RhoGAM is an injection of antibodies to the Rh factor that prevents isoimmunization in nearly 100 percent of cases. The antibodies in RhoGAM bind to the Rh protein on the fetal blood cells and "hide" them, blocking the mother's immune response. Before the development of RhoGAM in the 1960s, 50 percent of babies born to Rh negative mothers were stillborn.

If you are Rh negative, your partner can have his blood type checked. If he is also negative, your baby will be, too, and you do not need RhoGAM. If he is Rh positive, you can have a blood test done in the first trimester that can determine the Rh status of the baby.

RhoGAM is given to all Rh-negative mothers at twenty-eight weeks, and repeated after delivery if the baby is Rh positive. RhoGAM cannot cross the placenta, so there is no risk to the baby. It does not contain the mercury-based preservative thimerasol and poses no side effects for the mother.

Complete Blood Count (CBC)

A complete blood count is done to check for signs of infection, anemia, and blood-clotting problems.

Chlamydia and Gonorrhea (CT and GC)

A urine test or vaginal swab is used to screen for chlamydia and gonorrhea because these sexually transmitted diseases can cause eye infections in the newborn.

Hepatitis B

A blood test looks for the presence of hepatitis B, a viral liver infection. If a mother passes this virus to her baby during childbirth, the baby will likely become a carrier of the infection. As a carrier, the child can develop liver failure or cancer. Although hepatitis B is passed through bodily fluids, you can safely have a vaginal birth if you have hepatitis. A medication, hepatitis B immunoglobulin, given to the baby immediately after delivery, prevents the baby from becoming infected.

Human Immunodeficiency Virus (HIV)

There are fifty thousand new infections of HIV per year in the United States. A blood test for HIV is offered to all pregnant women. With the use of antiviral drugs during pregnancy and delivery, the risk of transmitting HIV to a baby is less than 1 percent. Women with active HIV should deliver by cesarean and should not breastfeed.

Human Papilloma Virus (HPV)

Testing for HPV is recommended routinely for all women over the age of thirty. If it is time for your regular Pap smear during pregnancy, an HPV test will be done as well. HPV is a sexually transmitted infection that causes cervical cancer and precancerous changes on the cervix. Nearly 85 percent of women (and men) will have this infection during their lifetime. For most women exposed to HPV, nothing ever happens. But a small number will develop precancerous cells on the cervix, which need to be monitored closely or removed.

HPV will not affect your baby in any way. You can still have a vaginal delivery. In fact, many women with precancerous cells on the cervix will find the problem has resolved after delivery because the abnormal cells are shed off during trauma of the birthing process.

Pap Smear

A Pap smear (a screening test for cervical cancer) should be done on all women starting at age twenty-one, and repeated every one to three years, depending on her risk factors. Prenatal visits are an excellent opportunity to have this screening test done if you have not had it done recently. The Pap smear is collected by brushing the cervix and is perfectly safe in pregnancy.

Rapid Plasma Reagin (RPR)

RPR is a blood test for syphilis—a sexually transmitted infection. If a woman has syphilis during pregnancy, it can cause congenital syphilis syndrome, which is associated with miscarriage, neurologic problems, and stillbirth. Women can be treated with antibiotics (usually penicillin), which is safe in pregnancy. About 100,000 women are diagnosed with syphilis every year in the United States.

Rubella

Rubella (also known as the German measles) is a viral infection that can cause birth defects and stillbirth. In the United States, most people are vaccinated for rubella as children. However, some women haven't been vaccinated or their immunity has worn off over time. During pregnancy, a blood test will determine whether you are immune to rubella. If you are not immune, you should avoid contact with people who may carry rubella. Thankfully, rubella has essentially been eliminated from the Western Hemisphere. In developing countries, nearly 25 percent of the population has not been adequately vaccinated. Pregnant women are not immune to rubella and who are traveling to developing countries or have contact with unvaccinated immigrants should take precautions. They should wash their hands frequently, make sure that children and close contacts have been vaccinated, and avoid contact with other people with illness and rashes. Pregnant women cannot be vaccinated during pregnancy because the rubella vaccine contains a live virus that can infect the baby.

The last epidemic of rubella in the United States was in 1964. Over 12 million people contracted the virus, resulting in 11,000 stillbirths and 20,000 birth defects.

Urine Culture

Your doctor will test your urine for the presence of a bladder infection, also known as a urinary tract infection (UTI). If you are found to have a UTI, you will be given an antibiotic that is safe in pregnancy. If a UTI is untreated, it can spread to the kidneys and can cause preterm labor.

Maternal Genetic Tests

As scientists discover the details of the human genome, screening for more than three thousand genetic disorders can be done. Genetic carrier testing involves a blood test to identify gene mutations that can be passed to a fetus. For a baby to be affected, both the mother and father must carry the mutation. Initially, a mother will be tested; if she has any gene mutations, her partner will then be tested. The most common autosomal recessive diseases are cystic fibrosis, Tay-Sachs disease, Gaucher's disease, and Canavan disease. Testing can be done before or during the pregnancy.

ACOG's Recommended Maternal Screenings

If a specific genetic disorder runs in your family, you will be offered a blood test to see whether you carry a gene mutation for that disease. If there are no known disorders, you will be screened based on your ethnic background:

All ethnicities: cystic fibrosis, spinal muscular atrophy

Eastern European Jewish/Ashkenazi: Tay-Sachs disease, familial dysautonomia, Canavan disease

African/Mediterranean/Southeast Asian: thalassemia, sickle cell disease

Benefits of testing: Carrier testing allows women to understand how their personal genetic makeup can influence their children. If you find out that your child has a genetic disorder, you can educate yourself about what to expect and identify specialists in your area before the baby is born. You may also choose to terminate the pregnancy.

Disadvantages of testing: Genetic testing is expensive, with tests costing $100 to $3,000. Insurance coverage varies widely by carrier. While a gene mutation may be identified, the effects of that mutation are not always known, which can lead to undue stress in a family. At this time, gene mutations cannot be corrected and the only alternative is pregnancy termination.

Personal choice: Genetic carrier testing is optional. Before having any tests done, you need to ask yourself some very personal questions. How significant is the disease you are testing for? What are your feelings about having a child with a chronic illness? Would a child with a genetic disorder be a heavy burden for your family? Your answers to these questions are not right or wrong. But they may guide you in deciding whether you want to do testing at all.

Fetal Genetic Tests

Each cell in our body contains twenty-three pairs of chromosomes, forty-six chromosomes in total. Chromosomes are made of DNA, which programs our characteristics, such as hair color, height, and risks for disease. We inherit one chromosome of each pair from our mother and one from our father.

Many families ponder what their baby will look like, whether it will be smart, or whether it will inherit its grandmother's curly hair. While these questions are fun to think about, what most patients really want to know is whether their baby will be "normal" or "healthy." Fetal genetic tests are done once you are pregnant to identify chromosomal disorders, such as extra or missing chromosomes, and birth defects related to the formation of the baby's spine and brain called neural tube defects (NTDs), such as spina bifida and anencephaly. Many women choose to keep their pregnancy secret from family and friends until they know the results of these tests.

The most common of these disorders is Down syndrome, in which there is an extra chromosome 21, also referred to as trisomy 21. Although women who are older than thirty-five are at the highest risk for these disorders, they can occur at any maternal age. In fact, more women under age thirty-five have babies with Down syndrome simply because more women under thirty-five give birth. Other chromosomal disorders that can be identified include trisomies 13, 18, 16, and 22, and Turner's syndrome (in which there is a missing X chromosome).

Chromosome abnormalities occur more frequently in older mothers (over age 35) because their eggs are more likely to be genetically abnormal. Women are born with all the eggs they will have, each initially containing forty-six chromosomes. At the time of ovulation, the egg divides in half, so it has only twenty-three chromosomes. Older eggs make mistakes in this process so that some eggs have an extra chromosome, while others are missing a chromosome. If one of these abnormal eggs is fertilized with sperm, the fetus will have a chromosomal abnormality. At age forty, over 90 percent of a woman's eggs are genetically abnormal. Millions of sperm, on the other hand, are newly generated every day and do not carry the chromosome abnormalities as frequently as eggs.

Fetal genetic testing takes two forms: screening tests and diagnostic tests. A screening test tells you the likelihood that your baby could have a birth defect; a diagnostic test tells you with more than 99 percent certainty whether the baby has the disorder. Screening tests are generally offered to women under age thirty-five and diagnostic tests are offered to women over age thirty-five.

Screening Tests

Screening tests are conducted to assess the chance that your baby has a particular condition. The test may suggest that your baby is at increased risk for a disorder when it is actually completely normal, known as a false-positive. In addition, a negative screening test does not guarantee that your baby is normal, known as a false-negative. Since screening tests only involve blood tests and ultrasounds, they pose no risk to the baby.

Integrated screening: Integrated screening for trisomies 21, 13, and 18 and for neural tube defects has three parts: a blood test in the first trimester, an ultrasound in the first trimester, and a blood test in the second trimester. Hormones produced by the pregnancy are measured in the mother's blood in the first trimester to identify specific patterns that are more common in babies with chromosomal disorders. The ultrasound measures the thickness of the skin behind the fetus's neck. Thicker skin has been associated with chromosome abnormalities. The third part, the blood test in the second trimester, measures alpha fetoprotein (AFP), which is a marker for neural tube defects. Integrated screening detects 95 percent of babies with Down syndrome, 90 percent of babies with trisomy 18, and 80 percent of trisomy 13 and neural tube defects.

Cell-free DNA testing: Cell-free DNA testing (cfDNA), also known as noninvasive prenatal testing (NIPT), is a blood test that can be done as early as nine weeks to detect fragments of fetal DNA in the mother's blood. Although fetal and maternal circulations do not mix, in 1997, scientists discovered pieces of a Y chromosome in a pregnant woman's blood. Initially, cell-free DNA testing was only used to determine the gender and blood type of a fetus. Now, it detects trisomies 21, 13, and 18. Some labs also test for Trisomy 16 and 22, as well as specific gene mutations. It does not detect neural tube defects.

The accuracy of this test depends on the amount of fetal DNA isolated, called the fetal fraction. The fetal fraction is influenced by the mother's weight, the gestational age, and sample collection methods. If the test is done very early or the mother is overweight, there may not be enough fetal DNA to determine a result. In these cases, another sample can be drawn later in the pregnancy.

In 2015, ACOG recommended that cfDNA be used only by patients who:

- Are age thirty-five and older
- Have had a chromosomal abnormality in a previous pregnancy
- Have an abnormal fetal ultrasound
- Have a positive integrated screening test

Cell-free DNA testing is being studied for use in low-risk women (under age thirty-five) and in twin pregnancies. The accuracy of the test appears to be similar to that for high-risk women.

Because cfDNA is a screening test, all abnormal results should be confirmed with a diagnostic test, such as amniocentesis. The test detects 99 percent of babies with trisomy 21 or 18, 85 percent of trisomy 13 and sex chromosome abnormalities, and is accurate in detecting gender in 98 percent. cfDNA costs between $1,200 and $1,800. Insurance covers cfDNA for women considered high risk. Some plans will also cover it for low-risk, younger women.

the doctor's diary

The cell-free DNA (cfDNA) test is one of the most significant advances in obstetrics in many years. Previously, women had to choose between the integrated screening—with its false positives and negatives, and amniocentesis—with its risk of miscarriage. The integrated screening looks at patterns of hormones, not at the DNA of the baby. Its results can be confusing for many patients who are accustomed to black and white answers. Many women are hesitant to have an amniocentesis, mostly because they are afraid they will miscarry. In addition, the amniocentesis can't be done until sixteen weeks, well into the second trimester when a woman is already showing.

The cfDNA test is a great alternative. It is a simple blood test, so it doesn't have any risks; it can be done as early as nine weeks; and its accuracy is very close to that of the amniocentesis for high-risk pregnancies (for women age thirty-five and older). Overall, it has the highest detection rate of the screening tests.

However, cfDNA testing differs from amniocentesis in a few ways and is not a substitute for it. The cfDNA test screens only for gender and the most common trisomies, so it won't pick up rare disorders that an amniocentesis will. It works best in high-risk women—unlike the amniocentesis that has the same accuracy no matter what your age. It can be done in the first trimester with plenty of time for further testing if necessary. While the cfDNA test doesn't guarantee that your baby is perfect, it is a great way to get information early without the fear of causing a miscarriage. Talk to your provider and see whether cfDNA is an option for you.

Diagnostic Tests

A diagnostic test looks directly at fetal chromosomes in a profile called a karyotype. The chromosomes are obtained by removing cells from the pregnancy itself. Diagnostic tests are considered nearly 100 percent accurate.

Chorionic villi sampling (CVS): CVS is a biopsy of the placenta done between eleven and thirteen weeks. The chorionic villi are fingerlike projections of the placenta that contain numerous blood vessels. They are bathed in maternal blood and are the place where nutrients pass from mother to baby. The biopsy is done by inserting a thin tube through the cervix and into the uterus, or it can also be taken through the abdomen with a needle. The risk of miscarriage as a result of this test is 1 in 100, and the cost of the test is $3,000.

Amniocentesis: Fetal skin and lung cells are found in amniotic fluid. An amniocentesis is a procedure by which an ob-gyn (usually a perinatologist) inserts a needle through the skin of the abdomen and into the amniotic sac. A small amount of amniotic fluid is withdrawn, and the fetal cells are isolated and sent to the lab for karyotype evaluation. This procedure can be done between fifteen and twenty-two weeks, has a risk of miscarriage of 1 in 300, and costs $2,000.

Choosing Fetal Genetic Testing

Like maternal carrier screening, fetal testing is optional. You may feel pressured to do these tests, especially if you are over age thirty-five. Deciding whether to do testing requires asking yourself what you would do with the information. If you would continue the pregnancy regardless of the results, it may not be worth it to do the test, especially if it carries a risk of miscarriage. You should clarify with your doctor what a "normal" result means. These tests only look for a few specific diseases, not every possible disease. Remember that your child's chromosomes cannot be corrected, so none of these diseases can be cured. However, you have the option to terminate the pregnancy. You can also use this information to prepare yourself and your family for taking care of a special-needs child.

Most patients look forward to getting their test results, assuming that they will be normal. But when the results are abnormal, more tests must be done. Waiting for test results and follow-up appointments can be very stressful. If you begin with the integrated screening test at twelve weeks, you will receive the results at fourteen weeks. If your result is abnormal, you will schedule an appointment with a genetic counselor and a perinatologist. If you decide to proceed with an amniocentesis, which can be done at sixteen weeks, you will receive the results at eighteen weeks. Now six to eight weeks will have passed since you took your first test, all the while wondering whether your baby is healthy. You can use this seemingly endless waiting period to educate yourself about the possible outcomes so you are familiar with what may be found. Keep in mind that the majority of test results will confirm that your baby is perfectly healthy.

Diabetes Screening

Pregnant women are screened for gestational diabetes mellitus (GDM) because babies of diabetics can grow large, putting them at risk for having a difficult delivery or needing a cesarean. Gestational diabetes is treated with blood sugar monitoring, dietary changes, and sometimes insulin.

Testing for GDM between twenty-four and twenty-eight weeks involves a blood sugar challenge, called the glucola test, in which you drink a solution containing 50 grams of glucose, followed by a blood test one hour later. Normally, the hormone insulin moves sugar out of the bloodstream and into cells. If your insulin levels are low or your cells are resistant to insulin, as is the case in diabetes, sugar remains in the blood longer. If your screening glucola test is high, you will undergo a second test. This test, called the 3-hour glucose tolerance test, first checks your blood sugar while fasting. Then, you drink 100 grams of a glucose solution and have blood tests at one, two, and three hours after the drink. The diagnosis of GDM is made if two or more results are abnormal.

Most providers screen all pregnant women for diabetes, while some may only test those with risk factors, such as having a family history of diabetes, being overweight, or being older than thirty-five. However, half of women with GDM do not have any of these risk factors.

The side effects of the screening glucola test, all due to rapid sugar intake, are nausea, dizziness, and headaches, which usually resolve within an hour. Some have questioned whether the ingredients in the drink are toxic. However, it has been used by millions of women over decades with no ill effects, apart from the risks cited here.

If you choose not to use the glucola test, you can monitor your blood sugar levels with a glucometer. You would check your blood sugar while fasting and one hour after meals for one week. Your provider may also allow you to substitute other foods that contain 50 grams of glucose—such as two slices of bread and one banana, twenty-eight jellybeans, or ten Twizzler strawberry twists—for the glucola drink.

Ultrasounds

Ultrasounds send pulsing sound waves from a transducer into the body. As the sound waves reflect back from the tissues, they are made into a picture. Ultrasound, which has been used for medical purposes since the 1950s, does not contain radiation like that found in X-rays or CT scans. The sound waves cannot be heard by the fetus because the frequency of waves from the ultrasound (1,000,000 hertz) is well above the range that can be heard by the human ear (20–20,000 hertz).

Ultrasound is one of the most commonly used tools in obstetrics. It can determine the gestational age of the pregnancy, see how many babies you have, identify birth defects, and help doctors estimate the fetal weight. However, ultrasounds cannot guarantee that your baby is healthy. They only detect anatomic birth defects, such as a malformation of the heart or a swelling in the kidney. They cannot be used to diagnose a chromosomal abnormality or a gene mutation. Even in the best of hands, 20 percent of anatomic abnormalities are missed.

The safety of ultrasounds has been well established. A review of over fifty medical studies shows that ultrasounds do not pose any danger to moms or fetuses. They do not cause birth defects, childhood developmental or intellectual problems, or cancer. Skeptics point to animal models in which an increase in fetal temperature from the ultrasound waves has been related to birth defects. However, for these defects to occur, the temperature would need to increase by at least 1.5 degrees, which would require over four hours of continuous ultrasound exposure. It is unlikely that the routine ultrasounds done during pregnancy—which last fifteen minutes or less—could cause harm. These findings from animal models have never been seen in humans. However, while there is no evidence of harm in humans, there is no evidence that no harm is possible. Therefore, doctors recommend having ultrasounds only when they are medically indicated.

During pregnancy, most women receive an ultrasound in the first trimester to confirm the gestational age and another one at twenty weeks, usually by a perinatologist, to look for birth defects. Ninety-eight percent of mothers receive at least one ultrasound, 70 percent have three or more, and 23 percent have six or more.[1]

This technology was originally designed to help doctors evaluate pregnancies with complications; it is now used universally. However, screening all pregnant women with ultrasound has never been shown to improve perinatal outcome when compared with patients who had ultrasounds only because of the presence of complications. Routine ultrasound in low-risk pregnancies does not decrease the risk of stillbirth, preterm birth, or other pregnancy complications, but leads to more medical interventions.[2]

An individual ultrasound costs $150 to $600. But because each mother receives a few, the cost of this test tops $1 billion per year. Most insurance carriers cover ultrasounds, but some consider them medically unnecessary and require the patient to pay out of pocket.

the doctor's diary

Ultrasounds have become commonplace. While patients think it is fun to see the baby—and it may be a great bonding experience—multiple ultrasounds do not improve the health of the pregnancy. Most ultrasound findings are not significant, and if the baby has anatomical defects, they cannot be corrected anyway. Many patients do not fully understand the purpose and limitations of an ultrasound and are falsely reassured that their baby is "perfect." Some women expect to see their baby on the ultrasound at every prenatal visit. I've even had patients leave my practice because they were disappointed that I wasn't going to "show" them the baby each time they came in.

For some mothers, having multiple ultrasounds instills fears about their pregnancy: the baby looks too big, the baby looks too small, the baby has the cord around its neck (actually a normal finding). Or maybe there was just "limited visualization," meaning some of the organs couldn't be evaluated completely because of the size or position of the baby. In the mom's mind, this translates to "there may be a problem."

Over the years I have seen a shift in doctors' philosophy about the health of a baby. In the past, a baby was presumed to be normal unless there was evidence to the contrary. Now a doctor feels that she needs to "prove" that the baby is healthy, and make sure her patients are receiving the most accurate information without missing anything significant. As a result, ultrasounds are often "overcalled" because doctors are afraid of missing something or want to recheck if something isn't clear—prompting more visits and ultrasounds. I have encountered some perinatologists in my community who always find something irregular on an ultrasound. They insist that they need to take another look, generating fear in the mother and increasing health-care costs.

Ultrasounds allow women to connect to their babies. Mothers love getting photographs of ultrasound pictures that make their baby "real" and sharing them with family members and friends. But some old-fashioned ways of bonding are great, too. Just sitting quietly and feeling your baby move first thing in the morning, having your partner talk to the baby with hands on your belly to feel the movements, and taking pictures of your growing belly every month to document the changes are all significant ways to connect to your baby.

3-D and 4-D Ultrasound

In addition to the standard ultrasound, 3-D and 4-D images are also available. A normal ultrasound gives a picture in two dimensions—length and width—in black and white, whereas 3-D ultrasound provides the third dimension—depth—in color as a still image. A 4-D ultrasound adds the final component—movement. These methods of imaging are mostly for novelty and entertainment, and aren't medically necessary. Insurance usually doesn't cover them so most women pay for them personally, at a cost of around $100.

the doctor's diary

Most families like to see a 3-D ultrasound so they can see their baby's face. However, it's rare to see a picture that looks like the ones in the advertisements. Most of the time, the baby has its face pressed against something, like the wall of the uterus, so it is difficult to make out any specific features. And I have to say—every baby in those photos looks exactly the same to me!

Cervical Exams

A cervical exam assesses the dilation and effacement of your cervix. During pregnancy, this exam is integral in making the diagnosis of preterm labor. Contractions without cervical change are called Braxton Hicks (false labor); contractions with cervical change are preterm labor. Near the due date, cervical exams are also used to confirm whether a woman is in labor and to make sure that the baby is head down.

Many patients have cervical exams during the last month of pregnancy with the hope of predicting when labor will start. Unfortunately, the cervical exam doesn't provide the answer. Sometimes a woman will be dilated 3 cm and remain like that for weeks, or another will have a closed, firm cervix and deliver the same day.

The results of a cervical exam are reported as a Bishop score. The Bishop score takes into account five characteristics: cervical dilation, cervical effacement, cervical position, cervical consistency, and station of the fetal head.

Score	Dilation	Effacement	Position	Consistency	Station
0	closed	0%	posterior	firm	-3
1	1–2cm	0–40%	mid	medium	-2
2	3–4cm	50–80%	anterior	soft	-1, 0
3	5cm	100%			+1, +2

Calculating a Bishop score is only helpful for predicting whether an induction of labor will be successful. If the Bishop score is 8 or less, the chance that the induction won't work, and that a cesarean will then be required, is 32 percent whereas a score above 8 will usually result in a vaginal delivery. The Bishop score does not have anything to do with predicting when spontaneous labor will start, though many doctors use it for that purpose. Neither does the Bishop score tell you how quick or slow your labor will be.

Cervical exams can be uncomfortable and may provoke unnecessary worrying about when you will deliver. If you aren't dilated at all, you may feel discouraged. If you find out you are dilated, you may rush to make all the last minute preparations, only to find yourself waiting for weeks.

the doctor's diary

To be honest, I'm not sure why cervical exams are done routinely during the last month of pregnancy. Maybe a mom with a "ready" cervix is more likely to agree to be induced. Feeling as if it's going to happen any minute prompts some doctors and women to schedule a date to get it going. In my experience, doing a cervical exam every week only causes frustration in moms who don't see anything happening and anxiety in those who are afraid their baby is going to pop out at any moment.

Antepartum Testing

Antepartum testing (APT) includes a variety of examinations that seek to identify babies who are at increased risk for stillbirth or complications from low oxygen levels, such as cerebral palsy. While the use of antepartum testing is widespread, there is limited evidence that it improves newborn outcomes.

The theory behind antepartum testing is that when a fetus isn't receiving enough oxygen or nutrition, it will conserve energy by moving less or slowing its heart rate. Eventually, it will cease producing amniotic fluid and stop moving completely. These changes in move-ment, heart rate, and amniotic fluid can be used to predict stillbirth.

Although high-risk pregnancies have a higher rate of stillbirth, 40 percent of stillbirths occur in pregnancies with no risk factors. High-risk pregnancies—those in which the mother has a chronic condition, such as diabetes or high blood pressure, there has been poor fetal growth or decreased fetal movement, postterm pregnancy, or the mother who has had a previous stillbirth—may benefit from antepartum testing. However, APT will not identify a sudden cata-strophic event, such as a placental abruption (when the placenta sep-arates from the wall of the uterus) or a compressed umbilical cord.

If an antepartum test is abnormal, your doctor may recommend an induction of labor or a cesarean section. Since there are risks to these procedures, any abnormal test should be confirmed by a second.

Types of Antepartum Testing

If your doctor or midwife recommends one of these antepartum tests, be sure to ask why and what she is hoping to discover.

Nonstress Test (NST)

The nonstress test is the most common type of antepartum test-ing. NST's are typically done during the third trimester for high-risk pregnancies. In the NST, a Doppler ultrasound is placed over the abdomen and secured with a belt. The fetal heart rate is measured and recorded continuously over a period of twenty to thirty minutes.

The fetal heart rate is not a steady number but rather varies between 120 and 160 beats per minute. The more variation of the heart rate within this range, the healthier the fetus. A heart rate that doesn't fluctuate may be the result of a lack of oxygen.

If the NST is normal, you can be assured that your baby is thriv-ing inside the womb. However, if the NST is abnormal, there is still a 60 percent chance that your baby is perfectly healthy.

Biophysical Profile (BPP)

The BPP looks at five indicators of fetal well-being via an ultrasound: the NST, breathing, body movements, tone, and amniotic fluid level. Each of these five indicators is given a score of 2 for normal and 0 for abnormal. If the total score is 8 or more, the risk for stillbirth is very low. If the score is 4 or less, the risk of stillbirth is 30 percent. If the score is 6, the test should be repeated in the next few days.

The BPP is done during the third trimester for high-risk women. The score can be affected by fasting; if the mother hasn't eaten in ten to twelve hours before the test, the result may be artificially low. If your doctor recommends a BPP, be sure you are well fed before you go!

Contraction Stress Test (CST)

The CST is also used for high-risk pregnancies to determine whether the fetus is receiving enough oxygen. For this test, intravenous Pitocin is given to stimulate contractions. If the baby's heart rate drops after a contraction, it is considered a positive test. However, like the NST, with a positive CST, there is a 50 percent chance that your baby is perfectly healthy.

Umbilical Artery Doppler Surveillance

A Doppler exam (ultrasound) of the umbilical artery evaluates the circulation of blood through the umbilical cord from the placenta to your baby. If the placenta is not working well, the blood does not flow normally. This test is used in cases of poor fetal growth. If the blood flow is significantly compromised, your doctor may recommend delivering the baby.

Fetal Movement/Kick Counts

A fetus begins to move at seven to eight weeks of pregnancy. However, because of the surrounding amniotic fluid and the thick uterine wall muscle, most women don't feel movement until sixteen to twenty weeks.

Decreased fetal movement can be a sign of low oxygen levels. In fact, stillbirth is 60 times more common in women who report decreased fetal movement. Many mothers have a concern about the frequency of fetal movements at least once during pregnancy.

During the last half of pregnancy, a healthy fetus is active 30 percent of the time and spends 70 percent of its time asleep. When performing kick counts, a mother should feel ten discrete movements within two hours. Formal kick counting only needs to be done in high-risk pregnancies, but it is important for all mothers to be aware of fetal movements and to notice any significant changes in the patterns.

Babies actually move much more often than a mother will feel. A movement seen on an ultrasound is perceived by the mother only half of the time. Fetal movement increases throughout the day, peaks late in the evening between nine p.m. and one a.m., and decreases in the middle of the night as maternal blood sugar levels fall.

If a baby isn't moving, it could be due to inadequate oxygen but more likely, it is related to the mother's perception of movement. You will feel less movement if:

- You are sitting or standing instead of lying down.
- You are distracted.
- The placenta is attached to the front wall of the uterus.
- The amniotic fluid is low.
- The fetus is positioned with its arms and legs toward the mother's back.
- You are overweight or obese.

A baby moving infrequently can be a cause for concern, but doctors are unsure of the significance of a baby who seems to move too much. Generally, doctors reassure patients that frequent strong movements and hiccups are not a reason to worry. However, a single episode of vigorous activity has been associated with stillbirth.[3] Any notable change should be reported to your provider.

Group B Streptococcus (GBS) Screening

Group B Streptococcus (GBS), also known as *Streptococcus agalactiae*, is a bacteria that lives in the vagina and intestines of 20 to 30 percent of women. The first cases of newborn infection were documented in 1964. By the 1970s, GBS was identified as the leading cause of newborn infections, with nearly half of infected babies dying. Before pregnant women were routinely screened for GBS, there were 8,500 cases of newborn GBS infections per year. With screening and treatment of women with GBS, the number of cases has declined to 2,000 per year. If you are found to carry GBS, you will be treated with antibiotics during labor to prevent the spread to the baby.

Screening of all pregnant women is done at thirty-five to thirty-seven weeks with a vaginal and rectal swab that is sent to a lab for a culture. Test results are available in forty-eight hours. Studies have shown that screening at this time most accurately predicts a woman's GBS status when she will enter labor over the next five weeks.

An alternative to the culture is a rapid test that looks for the bacteria's DNA. Results are usually available within two hours. However, this test is more expensive and less accurate than the culture. It can be done on a woman in labor if her GBS culture results are not available.

You can test positive for GBS at one time in the pregnancy, and negative at another. If you have ever tested positive in this pregnancy or a previous one, you are considered positive. In addition, if you have had a previous baby with GBS infection or GBS has been found in your urine, you should be treated while in labor. (See more about GBS treatment on page 253.)

Bed Rest

Approximately 20 percent of all pregnant women are prescribed bed rest for some period of time. There's "strict" bed rest and "modified" bed rest, both with arbitrary lists of dos and don'ts. Nearly all obstetricians admit to using bed rest as a treatment for pregnancy complications. While this seems like a simple therapy on the surface, it is incredibly difficult to adhere to and studies don't support its use for any complication of pregnancy.

Bed rest has been used in pregnancy for hundreds of years. Historically, in some cultures, women with seemingly normal pregnancies were separated from society for the last month of gestation, a situation called confinement. Even now, we still refer to the due date as the EDC (estimated date of confinement).

Despite a plethora of medical evidence refuting its value, women are put on bed rest for a variety of conditions in pregnancy, including elevated blood pressure, preterm labor, cervical incompetence, placenta previa, prevention of miscarriage, twins, and poor fetal growth. In a review of seventeen complications of pregnancy for which bed rest was prescribed, there were no benefits whatsoever in the outcomes for the babies. The Society for Maternal-Fetal Medicine has gone so far as to say that prescribing bed rest to pregnant women in any situation is "unethical."[4] Yet it continues to be done regularly. The cost of bed rest, including in-hospital care, doctors' visits, loss of wages, and the cost to hire help around the house, is estimated to be a staggering $1.6 billion per year.

Bed rest has its own inherent risks:

- Blood clots: The risk of developing a blood clot during pregnancy is 1 per 1,000. If you are on bed rest, the risk increases 16-fold.
- Weakened muscles and thinner bones
- Financial stress from leaving work
- Depression and anxiety
- Weight loss
- Preterm delivery

I am amazed at how many mothers are put on bed rest. We prescribe it because we simply have nothing else to offer. Women follow the advice because they want to feel like they are doing "something" in an otherwise desperate situation. But I believe that we are doing our patients a disservice by suggesting bed rest, and giving patients hope that we can fix something that we can't.

If your doctor recommends bed rest, you should make sure that you understand why. It is acceptable to question your doctor's advice and be clear about the goals of bed rest and how it would help you. If the idea of activity restriction makes you stressed, it may actually do more harm than good. You can even explain to your doctor that you have researched the topic and found that bed rest may not be helpful. As more patients question this outdated recommendation, clinical practice may eventually change. Perhaps raising awareness about this topic will spare future generations of women from weeks of lying in bed.

❧ TONYA'S STORY ❧

Tonya was a new associate at her law firm. She was working long hours and packing her weekends with activities. Petite, fit, and athletic, she was thrilled to find out she was pregnant and wanted to maintain her normal activities during her pregnancy. Everything was going well until about twenty-eight weeks. At her routine visit, her OB noticed that her fundal height measured a little small at 26 cm. Tonya had gained almost 20 pounds at this point, but still looked as if she could be only twenty weeks, with her small frame and tight abdominal muscles. To be on the safe side, her OB sent her to a perinatologist for an ultrasound. At that visit, the course of Tonya's pregnancy changed dramatically. The perinatologist said that the baby measured small and that Tonya needed to stop work immediately and stay on strict bed rest for the rest of the pregnancy. He counseled her that she could get out of bed to fix her meals and use the bathroom, but otherwise needed to stay put.

Tonya broke the news to her firm, who seemed understanding. Yet, because she was in the midst of an important case, she worried that her absence would influence her chances of becoming a partner someday. She lay in bed day in and day out. She went for ultrasounds every two weeks. The doctor continually put fear in her mind about her baby's size. She asked whether the baby's size could be normal—because she was petite herself. Tonya felt that the doctor dismissed her questions. She was encouraged to stick with the bed-rest program.

As a result of her ten weeks of bed rest, Tonya suffered from back pain, insomnia, and depression. She tried to tell herself it would be worth it—because she would do anything for her baby.

At thirty-eight weeks, her doctor told her that she needed to be induced and that the baby would be better on the outside. She trusted his judgment, although she had been hoping for a more natural experience. At thirty-eight weeks, she had a vaginal birth of a 7 pound 9 ounce girl—slightly larger than average size.

Tonya has no regrets about the course of her pregnancy but questioned whether she really needed the bed rest. Although she wondered if her baby was small because she, herself was small, she never thought to ask the doctor whether bed rest was proven to be a benefit for women with "small babies." She trusted what he said completely. 🍃

During pregnancy, you will be offered many tests and interventions. By understanding the purpose and limitations of these examinations, you will be better equipped to make a decision about which you should do. Some tests give powerful information that makes your pregnancy safer and healthier. Others only lead to more tests, and the stress that accompanies them. If a particular action doesn't make sense to you, let your provider know your concerns. These are all personal decisions, but through communication with your provider, you can make the best choice together.

EXPECTING THE UNEXPECTED

—Pregnancy Risks and Complications

the doctor's diary

After twenty years in this business, I can tell you that being an obstetrician is never boring. I have taken care of thousands of women, each of them with a unique story. While it may sound clichéd, no two pregnancies are alike. Even patients who are completely healthy and have natural births will take away something different from the experience. I can't recall how many times I have heard a patient say that her pregnancy and especially her birth were far different from what she had imagined.

MOST WOMEN BEGIN THEIR PREGNANCY ASSUMING THAT EVERYthing will be normal and follow a predictable course. But the unexpected can happen. Over half of all pregnancies become "high risk," requiring interventions such as additional doctors' visits, ultrasounds, bed rest, or even cesareans. An unforeseen complication for you or your baby may lead you away from your desired plans.

However, if you learn about some of the more common challenges, you will be prepared for whatever comes your way.

The Risks of Being an Older Mother

Obviously, age is not a complication per se, but it does impact the course of your pregnancy. Biologically and physically, the best time for pregnancy and birth may be when a woman is in her early to midtwenties. This is when she rarely has medical problems, her body is strong, and her eggs are healthy. However, if you take into account social and economic factors, the best time to embark on motherhood may be when a woman is in her thirties. It appears that, in the developed world, humans mature reproductively about ten years before they mature socially, culturally, and financially. In the end, the decision to have a baby is based more on emotional and logistical factors than scientific ones, and varies from culture to culture, country to country, woman to woman.

the doctor's diary

Advanced maternal age (AMA)—oh, how I hate that term! No one wants to be put in the "old mother" category. But given that the other options are *elderly primigravida* or *geriatric mother*, which were common descriptions in the 1970s, I guess we are stuck with AMA. Technically, you are AMA if you are over thirty-five when you deliver. In the United States, 14 percent of all births are to women in this age group.

Here's the good news: most women over age thirty-five will have not have any problems with their pregnancy or delivery. Nonetheless, all older moms are technically considered high risk because their chance for a complication is higher than that of a younger woman. Other than smoking and drinking alcohol excessively, being over thirty-five influences the outcome of pregnancy more than any other factor. Studies show that even when patients with medical problems are excluded from the data, older mothers are more likely to have a miscarriage, need a cesarean, give birth to a small baby, or experience a stillbirth. But it is important to keep these risks in perspective. For example, the risk of having a baby with Down syndrome at age forty is 1 in 53; but that means that fifty-two of fifty-three mothers will have a genetically normal baby. The risk of stillbirth for mothers of advanced maternal age is 0.53 percent and 99.47 percent of babies will be perfectly safe.

Risks for the Older Mother

- Infertility: From age 35 to 40, the chance of conceiving is 10 percent per month. Over age 40, it decreases to 5 percent.
- Miscarriage: Older mothers have a higher chance of miscarriage.
  - *Ages 35–39:* The risk is 25 percent.
  - *Ages 40–44:* The risk is 51 percent.
  - *Age 45 and older:* The risk is 93 percent.
- Chromosomal abnormalities: At age 40, 90 percent of a woman's eggs are genetically abnormal. The risk of having a baby with Down syndrome, by age:
  - *Age 20:* 1 in 1,200
  - *Age 30:* 1 in 700
  - *Age 35:* 1 in 240
  - *Age 40:* 1 in 53
  - *Age 45:* 1 in 20
- Underlying medical problems: Women over age 35 are more likely to have diabetes and high blood pressure.
- Stillbirth: Older mothers have an increased chance of having a stillbirth. Most likely, this occurs because the blood vessels within the placenta are thicker and stiffer than

those seen in placentas of younger women. However, this risk is seen only in first-time mothers. The risk of stillbirth, by age:

- *Age 25–29:* 0.27 percent
- *Age 30–34:* 0.31 percent
- *Age 35–39:* 0.40 percent
- *Age 40 and older:* 0.53 percent

• Long labor: Prolonged labor is more common because the uterine contractions are not as effective or coordinated. In addition, the muscles and ligaments of the pelvis are less flexible, so a vaginal delivery can be more challenging, especially if a woman is having her first baby.

the doctor's diary

I often felt bad for my forty-year-old first-time moms. They would do everything right—read every book, ask lots of questions, take childbirth classes—and then would be stuck with a labor that went on for days. Meanwhile, my eighteen-year-old patient would not prepare at all, show up at the hospital knowing nothing about what was going to happen, and push the baby out in minutes.

————————

• **Cesareans:** Older mothers are more likely to deliver by cesarean because they have a higher chance of having a breech baby, obesity, diabetes, preeclampsia, and failure to progress in labor. This increased risk may also be related to physician's bias as well as the fact that older women tend to request elective cesareans more frequently.

The chance of a cesarean is:

- *Under age 25:* 23.6 percent
- *Ages 26–35:* 32.1 percent
- *Ages 35–39:* 40.8 percent
- *Age 40 and older:* 53.5 percent

There are pros and cons to having a baby at each age in a woman's life. While it may seem that the list of risks for older moms is ominous, waiting to have a baby may be the best decision for you. Maybe you want to pursue a career you love, or you didn't meet the right partner when you were young. You may want to be financially stable or have a home that could accommodate a family before you started one. Despite the risks of being a "geriatric mother," there are actually some advantages for your child. Children of older mothers have improved health and development compared to those of young mothers. They experience fewer injuries and have better language and social development. They also tend to get more attention from their parents and benefit from their parents' emotional and financial stability. There may never be a perfect time to become pregnant. You will likely always feel as if you need to be more settled, more financially secure—more "ready." But know that whatever age you are, your doctor or midwife will help you have the best outcome possible.

When Your Plans Change

A high-risk pregnancy is one that endangers the health of the mother or baby in some way. Sometimes the risks arise from health issues a woman has prior to becoming pregnant, such as high blood pressure or obesity. Some are related to behaviors and lifestyle choices, such as smoking and drinking alcohol. Others, such as having a breech baby or a placenta previa, seem to occur out of the blue. These unpredictable complications are the ones that frustrate patients and doctors the most. But just because something comes up in your pregnancy that you haven't anticipated, doesn't mean that you don't have options, or at least can prepare appropriately. You may need to let go of your original birth plan or other ideas about how your pregnancy will play out. The good news is that you can make adjustments with the guidance of your provider and still have the positive birth experience you want.

Breech Babies

The ideal position for a baby during a vaginal birth is head first, or *vertex presentation*. When a baby's head is at the top of the uterus, the baby is in breech presentation and its feet or buttocks will deliver first. Prior to twenty-eight weeks, many babies (28 percent) are breech. As the pregnancy progresses, most of these will naturally turn to the head-down position. At thirty-two weeks, 14 percent, and at thirty-six weeks, 9 percent are breech. By the due date, only 3 to 4 percent of babies are still in this position. Once a baby turns to vertex presentation, it usually stays in that position because its head fits more comfortably into the pelvis. If your baby hasn't turned by thirty-six weeks, it becomes less likely that it will. At this point, your provider will discuss options with you. Remember that over half of the babies who are breech in the last month will still turn spontaneously before birth.

Babies are more likely to stay in the breech position if your uterus has an unusual shape, the amniotic sac has too much or too little fluid, you are older, or your abdominal muscles and pelvic ligaments are unusually tight or loose. Having a placenta that is attached to the lowest part of the uterus or a short umbilical cord also hinders movement of the baby. Premature babies are breech more often because they haven't yet had time to turn.

Three Types of Breech

1. **Frank:** Butt down with legs straight (pike position) and feet near the head is the most common breech position.
2. **Complete:** Butt down with knees bent so the feet are near the buttocks.
3. **Footling, also known as incomplete:** One or both feet are below the buttocks. This is the most dangerous because cord prolapse (explained on page 151) is more likely.

If your baby is still breech at full term, you have three options: schedule a cesarean, attempt to turn the baby to vertex presentation, or deliver the baby vaginally. These days, most breech babies are born by cesarean.

Turning a Breech Baby

If your baby is breech, there are a variety of techniques you or your provider can use to turn the baby.

- Postures: There are certain positions that stretch and align the pelvis to encourage the baby to turn. These should be started at 34 weeks.
  - *Knees-to-chest position:* Kneel on the floor with your knees hip distance apart, rest your forehead and upper chest on floor, with your buttocks up in air, and hold the position for 15 minutes several times per day. If you can't get your chest on the floor, you can rest your forehead on a pillow.
  - *Pelvic tilt:* Lie on your back. Place a pillow under your hips so they are elevated 9 to 12 inches and you are at a 45-degree angle. Maintain this position for 15 minutes, 3 times per day.
- Webster technique: This is an adjustment done by a chiropractor to properly align the pelvis and stretch the ligaments to enlarge the space the baby has in which to turn.
- Moxibustion: This is a Chinese medicine technique in which the herb *Artemisia vulgaris* (mugwort) is burned near the little toe on each foot, which is an acupuncture point. Used in conjunction with acupuncture, this technique decreases the incidence of breech by 27 percent.[1]
- External cephalic version (ECV): This procedure, done in the hospital, is the manual rotation of the baby to the head-down position. ECVs are scheduled at 37 weeks so

that if there is a complication during the procedure, the baby can be delivered by cesarean and will not be premature. Prior to the procedure, the mother will have a saline lock placed so an IV can be connected should a cesarean be required. One or two doctors perform the ECV. A medication is given to relax the uterine muscle. The woman lies on her back in bed with one doctor on each side of the bed, sitting or standing. One doctor places both hands on the baby's head and the other places the hands on the butt. They will apply firm, constant pressure on the head and the butt in either a clockwise or counterclockwise direction. In this way, the baby will do a somersault—hopefully! After a few minutes of pressure, the doctor will check the fetal heart rate with ultrasound to confirm that the baby is tolerating the procedure. ECV is successful 58 percent of the time, especially if the mother has had children before, is at an earlier gestational age, has a posterior placenta, and has normal amniotic fluid volume.[2] ECV is less likely to be successful in women who are obese or those with tight abdominal muscles. Commonly, when the baby moves, its heart rate will drop temporarily, and return to normal once it has stabilized in its new position. Sometimes, however, the heart rate doesn't recover—especially if the cord has become wrapped around the baby. In those cases, an emergency cesarean will be performed. Despite the success rate of ECV, only 38 percent of women undergo this procedure.[3]

Risks of Vaginal Breech Delivery

The risks associated with a vaginal breech delivery are head entrapment and, if the baby is a footling breech, cord prolapse.

Birth was designed for the largest part—the head—to come out first. Head entrapment occurs when the baby's thinner body is delivered but the larger head gets stuck. When head entrapment oc-curs, the umbilical cord becomes compressed and the baby doesn't receive enough oxygen.

Cord prolapse is a dangerous condition in which the umbilical cord slips past the baby and through the open cervix. Normally, the baby's head or buttocks prevents this from happening. If a baby has one or both of its feet near the birth canal, the cord can slip past the baby into the vagina. When the cord is in the birth canal, it can easily be compressed, compromising the oxygen supply to the baby. A breech baby is twenty times more likely to have a cord prolapse than is one that is vertex.

The chance that a baby will die from a complication of a vagi-nal vertex delivery or cesarean is 0.5 per 1,000. In comparison, the chance with a vaginal breech delivery is 3 per 1,000, six times higher. If the breech delivery is attempted at home, the mortality rate is even greater, 22 per 1,000—44 times higher than a cesarean.[4]

the doctor's diary

I have only delivered three breech babies vaginally in my entire career and have done only one in the last fifteen years. By the time I started residency in 1995, malpractice lawsuits brought as a consequence of breech deliveries were becoming common. My first breech delivery was when I was an intern and had been on the job for just a few months. Back then, we would use X-rays to measure the size of the mother's pelvic bones to determine whether her pelvis was large enough to allow a breech delivery. An intern would always accompany the patient when she went to the radiology department for the X-rays.

On one of my trips to radiology in the middle of the night, I helped my patient move to the X-ray table as we waited for the technician to take the pictures. My patient was breathing heavily and looked distressed, al-though she never made a sound. I noticed that there was a large amount of bloody mucus on the sheets. I put on a pair of gloves, and found that the baby was ready to deliver, butt first! I told her that she could push if she wanted to. She gave a gentle push and the baby's body was de-livered to its shoulders. I reached a finger up its chest to free one arm, then the other. I kept the neck flexed as she pushed one last time and the head was out. I stood there, alone with her, in the cold radiology department, as her baby took its first breath. I remember thinking how simple and easy this birth had been.

Despite my impressive first breech birth, today I do not feel comfortable with vaginal breech deliveries because of my lack of experience. These deliveries require hands-on training as well as study. But because they are done so infrequently, it is difficult for any doctor or midwife to keep these skills sharp.

In the year 2000, one of the largest studies on the safety of vaginal breech delivery—the Term Breech Trial—concluded that a planned cesarean was significantly safer for the baby than was a vaginal birth.[5] Since then, most doctors don't give their patients any option other than a cesarean. Physicians who haven't delivered a breech baby vaginally in many years are no longer confident they have the necessary skills. Some younger doctors have never even seen a breech birth. From the doctor's perspective, delivering vaginally is not worth risking harm to the baby, criticism from colleagues, or a potential lawsuit if a complication arises.

If you have been planning for a natural birth and find out your baby is breech, you may feel disappointed. You need to find trusted information and understand all of your options. You may want to embark on a search for someone in your community who still performs vaginal breech deliveries or will help you to turn the baby.

the doctor's diary

There is no question that vaginal breech delivery is riskier than a vertex delivery. But the absolute risk is still low. This lost art needs to be taught in residency training so that the next generation of doctors feels comfortable with this option again. If more women request this alternative, doctors may be compelled to consider it. In addition, doctors and midwives should evaluate the position of the baby earlier in the pregnancy. Traditionally, they check the position at thirty-six weeks. But if they were to confirm that a baby was in breech position at thirty-two weeks, women would have more time to try some of the common turning techniques, such as practicing postures and moxibustion with acupuncture. When the baby is smaller, these techniques are more likely to be successful.

Doctors should encourage their patients to try an ECV. As stated earlier, only 38 percent of women undertake this option, but given its nearly 60 percent success rate, many cesareans could be averted.

If a Baby Won't Turn

If you have tried everything and your baby still won't turn, you may have no other option than a cesarean. As disheartening as this may be, it is a safer choice than having a vaginal breech birth with an inexperienced provider—and these days most providers are inexperienced. In the United States, accredited birthing centers don't allow breech deliveries, and some states, such as California, have laws prohibiting midwives from delivering breech babies at home. In time, if the number of skilled providers grows, the vaginal breech delivery may be a viable option again.

Diabetes (Gestational Diabetes Mellitus, or GDM)

Diabetes is a condition that affects the way the body processes blood sugar (glucose) so that sugar levels are abnormally high. Some women have diabetes before they become pregnant, but it can also arise as result of the pregnancy itself, known as gestational diabetes. The current recommendation is to screen all women for this condition between twenty-four and twenty-eight weeks. (See page 130 for details on this test.) Although gestational diabetes resolves once the baby is born, it increases the risk of developing overt diabetes in the next five to ten years. Women who have had GDM should follow up with their primary physician every two to three years for diabetes screening.

Insulin is a hormone made in the pancreas that moves glucose from the bloodstream into cells. Women with GDM are resistant to the effects of insulin and therefore their blood glucose levels remain high. The resistance to insulin is caused by a hormone, human placental lactogen (hPL). Science has yet to discover why one woman reacts to hPL by developing diabetes and another one doesn't. Although obesity, advanced maternal age, and a family history of diabetes increase the likelihood of developing GDM, many women have no risk factors.

Glucose is the main source of energy for the growing fetus. If a mother's blood sugar levels are persistently high, the baby will receive more sugar than it needs and, like us, will store the sugar as fat and grow excessively large. A large baby may have problems during delivery, such as a shoulder dystocia, or require a cesarean birth. After birth, large babies may experience other problems, such as difficulty breathing, jaundice, and low blood sugar. The fetus of a diabetic mother is accustomed to receiving lots of sugar from its mother. When the baby is born and no longer has a continuous sugar source, its blood sugar drops dramatically. Sometimes, this can be quite dangerous, leading to seizures. Therefore, newborns of diabetic mothers will have their blood sugar monitored closely. If the level is low, they will be given a sugar water solution or IV fluids to correct the condition.

Reducing the Chance of GDM

There are no guarantees, but there are some steps you can take to reduce your risk of developing gestational diabetes. Fetal growth is most influenced by glucose levels immediately after meals. Avoiding high spikes in blood sugar will help the fetus maintain a normal growth pattern. Starting in the second trimester, you should limit your intake of simple carbohydrates and increase your consumption of complex carbohydrates and protein. Simple carbohydrates—such as rice, white bread, and candy—cause blood sugar levels to rise rapidly, peak, and then decline; whereas complex carbohydrates—such as green vegetables, whole grains, and beans—and proteins are digested more slowly, and lead to a slower rise of blood sugar levels with a lower peak. In addition, women who exercise regularly before and during pregnancy can reduce their risk of developing gestational diabetes by 70 percent.[6] The effect is most significant when the exercise is vigorous.

Managing GDM

Women with GDM will be instructed to follow a special diet that includes complex carbohydrates and proteins, and to exercise regularly. They will monitor their blood sugar throughout the pregnancy with a machine called a glucometer. The testing is done first thing in the morning (before eating) as well as an hour after meals. The doctor will review the test results on a regular basis. If a woman has low to moderate insulin resistance, decreasing simple carbohydrates in the diet and exercising should be sufficient to keep her blood sugar levels normal. Women with GDM will also have extra ultrasounds during the third trimester, to monitor the growth of the baby. Most women who manage their GDM with diet and exercise alone and have good control of the blood sugar can wait for spontaneous labor and do not need to be induced.

If a woman's blood sugar levels are high despite dietary changes, she may need to take insulin. Women who are on insulin or who have poorly controlled diabetes should have labor induced at thirty-nine weeks because they have a higher chance of stillbirth. If the estimated fetal weight is greater than 4,500 grams (9 pounds 15 ounces), they will be offered a cesarean.

Treating diabetes decreases the chance of having a large baby and a shoulder dystocia by 50 percent. If you have GDM and are seeing a midwife for prenatal care, she will consult with an obstetrician as well. If your blood sugars are well controlled, she may still deliver your baby. If your blood sugars are out of the normal range, you should give birth in a hospital under the care of a doctor.

Hyperemesis

Most women (50 to 90 percent) experience nausea during the first trimester. In fact, it is the most common symptom of early pregnancy. However, some women (2 percent) go on to develop hyperemesis gravidarum, a severe form of morning sickness. These women have so much nausea and vomiting that they develop nutritional deficiencies, weight loss of at least 5 percent, dehydration, and metabolic imbalances.

It seems counterintuitive that a pregnant woman would become so nauseous during pregnancy that she can't keep food down. Records from the 1800s show that doctors thought toxins or infections were to blame. In the 1960s and 1970s, many believed it was a psychological disorder. Today, the cause is thought to be a reaction to elevated levels of estrogen and hCG (human chorionic gonadotropin) that accompany pregnancy.

Women are more likely to develop hyperemesis if they are carrying twins, have a history of nausea with birth control pill use, or have previously suffered from heartburn. Hyperemesis is also more common in women who are having their first baby and for those carrying a girl. While the condition may prevent you from eating normally, your fetus will continue to grow by taking whatever it needs from the vitamins and minerals stored in your body. Especially in the first trimester, the developing fetus is incredibly small, measuring only a few inches, and doesn't require many calories for growth.

Although hyperemesis is an uncomfortable and often miserable condition, with modern medication and treatment, severe complications are rare. Maternal mortality is virtually nonexistent. There is no difference in birth weight for babies born to mothers with hyperemesis, as long as the woman catches up with appropriate weight gain in the second half of her pregnancy. There is also no increase in birth defects in these babies.

Treatment: Coping with Hyperemesis

- Eat small meals of bland food: Food should be eaten slowly in small amounts every two hours to avoid overfilling the stomach. Fluids can be sipped through a straw and should be served cold. Women with hyperemesis most easily tolerate clear fluids that are carbonated and sour, such as those with lemon or lime flavoring.

- Avoid triggers: Strong odors, quickly changing positions, or spending too much time in heat and humidity may set off nausea.

- Watch your iron intake: Temporarily discontinue the use of iron supplements or prenatal vitamins with iron.

- Increase your activity: Exercise releases natural endorphins that ease nausea. Although lying in bed sounds much more appealing than going for a walk, physical activity will make you feel better.

- Try acupuncture or acupressure: Either one, used at the P6 site on the wrist, is a popular treatment, although a review of medical literature does not show a significant improvement in nausea. The P6 site is on the underside of the lower arm, three fingers-breadth from the bend in the wrist—where you can feel the tendon. You can also press on the site yourself or use seasickness bands sold over the counter at drugstores.

- Add ginger to your diet: Ginger can be taken raw, as capsules, lollipops, or tea. Research studies have shown that it improves the feeling of nausea. The dosage is 250 mg capsules four times per day.

- Take vitamin B_6: Studies support the use of vitamin B_6 (pyridoxine) for coping with nausea. The dosage is 25 mg three times per day.

- Try over-the-counter antihistamines: Doxylamine, an over-the-counter medication found in the brand-name sleep aids Unisom and Sominex, is also commonly used to treat nausea. It has been studied extensively for use in pregnancy and has been found safe and effective. However, it may have side effects, such as dry mouth and drowsiness, so is better used at night.

- Ask your doctor for a prescription medication: Your doctor can prescribe antiemetic drugs. Diclegis is a combination of vitamin B_6 and doxylamine, and is the only FDA-approved drug for the treatment of hyperemesis. While it is convenient to have both medications in one tablet, it is more expensive than purchasing the two drugs separately over the counter. Diclegis costs $575 for 100 tablets, whereas over-the-counter vitamin B_6 and generic doxylamine each cost about $10 for 100 tablets. Other drugs commonly used for hyperemesis are metoclopramide (Reglan) and ondansetron (Zofran). While these medications may be safe and effective, they have not been approved by the FDA for use in pregnancy.

- Use medical intervention: In extreme cases a woman can receive hydration or nutrition through an IV.

Intrauterine Growth Restriction (IUGR)

In 2015, Sarah Stage, a model, documented her pregnancy on Instagram. Even in the last month of pregnancy, Sarah's six-pack was still well defined. She received much criticism from the public that she wasn't eating enough and that she cared more about her looks than her baby. The critics were finally quieted when she gave birth to an 8 pound 7 ounce boy.

Thankfully, most women who look "small" during pregnancy have perfectly healthy babies. However, some fetuses don't grow well. Poor fetal growth is called intrauterine growth restriction (IUGR). IUGR is diagnosed when a baby's estimated weight is below the tenth percentile for that gestational age. Of course, some babies are simply genetically small. To distinguish a baby who is not growing well from one who is naturally small, your doctor will look for other ultrasound findings that are related to IUGR such as low amniotic fluid levels, diminished blood flow through the umbilical cord, and certain patterns of growth.

the doctor's diary

Many times in my career, I have found myself reassuring a woman after she has heard a remark from a stranger like, "How could you be due in a month? You're so tiny!" While some pregnant women would relish being called "small," most are unnerved if a well-meaning friend suggests that her baby isn't growing well. Some women even fib about their due date to deflect the commentary about how much more they need to eat, because they are not showing as much as others expect them to be.

Truth be told, no one can tell how big your baby is just by looking at you. There are many different factors that influence how your belly looks—from how tight your abs are to whether you've had a baby before. If people make negative comments about your size, let them know that your doctor or midwife is keeping an eye on things for you.

Causes of IUGR include:

- Fetal factors: Chromosomal abnormalities; birth defects; twins; infections, such as toxoplasmosis, chicken pox, syphilis, rubella, and CMV
- Placenta factors: Poor blood flow through the placenta or a separation of the placenta from the wall of the uterus
- Maternal issues: Diabetes, high blood pressure, mother's age greater than forty, uterine malformations, smoking, and alcohol use

At each prenatal visit after twenty weeks, your provider will measure the growth of your baby using a technique called fundal height. Fundal height is the measurement in centimeters from the pubic bone to the top of the uterus. The measurement corresponds to your baby's gestational age. The fundal height is most accurate if the same provider measures it at each visit. The measurements are compared from one visit to the next to confirm normal growth. If the fundal height and your gestational age do not match, it may be an indicator of IUGR. However, a discrepancy may also exist if your due date is wrong, your abdominal wall muscles are significantly tight, your baby is naturally small, or you are having your first baby.

Most babies (70 percent) diagnosed with IUGR have no significant problems after delivery. However, in severe cases, IUGR can cause bleeding in the fetal brain, cerebral palsy, problems with the lungs and intestines, and stillbirth. If your baby has IUGR, you should deliver with an ob-gyn in the hospital setting.

Treatment for IUGR

If your baby has been diagnosed with IUGR, you may continue with your normal activities. Such treatments as nutritional supplements, low-dose aspirin, and maternal oxygen have not been proven to correct the growth restriction. Bed rest at home or in the hospital is commonly recommended, but studies have shown that it does not improve outcomes. Ultrasounds are done every two to four weeks to measure the fetal growth.

An NST (nonstress test) will be done at least weekly. Babies with poor blood flow in the umbilical arteries may require daily monitoring. If your doctor determines that the baby's growth has stopped or that the blood flow through the placenta is severely compromised, he will recommend delivering the baby.

Macrosomia—Why Doctors Care So Much About "Big Babies"

Macrosomia describes a newborn weighing more than 4,500 grams (9 pounds 15 ounces). The diagnosis can only be made after delivery, but can be suspected during pregnancy. Macrosomia affects 5 to 10 percent of babies. Your baby may grow large if your previous baby was macrosomic, you have diabetes, you are overweight, you've gained more than the recommended amount of weight, you've passed your due date, you are carrying a boy, you were a large baby at birth, or you are tall.

Having a vaginal birth with a large baby poses risks to both the mother and fetus. For the mother, labor progresses slowly and may completely stall so that a cesarean is necessary. If the vaginal birth is successful, she may have a genital tract injury or excessive bleeding.

For the baby, there is a possibility for shoulder dystocia, low blood sugar at birth, and obesity in childhood. Of these, the most dangerous is shoulder dystocia, in which the head delivers but the shoulders get stuck. The nerves in the neck are overly stretched, which can lead to permanent paralysis of the arm and hand. In addition, if the dystocia is not relieved within minutes, the baby won't get enough oxygen and can have brain damage. For babies weighing over 4,500 grams, the risk of shoulder dystocia is 15 percent. If the mother is also diabetic, the risk climbs to 35 percent.

Doctors worry—some would even say obsess—about "big babies." Shoulder dystocia is unpredictable, unpreventable, and one of the most common reasons for malpractice lawsuits in obstetrics. Shoulder dystocia is more common with large babies, but it can also occur in routine deliveries with babies of normal size. Permanent injury to a baby may happen despite the best possible care. Ideally, if we knew the exact size of the baby before birth, we could better predict the risk of dystocia.

Many women have an ultrasound at the end of pregnancy to determine fetal weight. Ostensibly the ultrasound is looking for macrosomia. Ultrasounds use measurements from different body parts to estimate the weight. However, because fetuses are 3-dimensional, irregularly shaped, and of varying densities, a doctor's ability to predict weight using ultrasound is limited. The actual weight may be 10 to 20 percent larger or smaller than the estimate. A woman who has given birth previously is often able to estimate her baby's weight just as accurately as an ultrasound. One-third of mothers are told that they are having a "big baby." Of these, the average birth weight is 7 pounds 13 ounces—just 5 ounces more than the average size of a baby.

Many doctors will try to avoid shoulder dystocia altogether by recommending that any patient whose baby seems big should have an early induction or cesarean. However, the American College of Obstetricians and Gynecologists (ACOG) recognizes that inducing labor or doing a cesarean in these cases doesn't benefit the mother or baby in any way. Therefore, they insist that these procedures should not be done. Despite their recommendation, having a "big baby" is one of the most common reasons for induction and cesarean in the United States today.

the doctor's diary

If your doctor suggests that you have a "big baby," it is important not to panic. The estimated fetal weight is exactly that—an estimate. Most babies are perfectly designed to fit their mothers. Having a "big baby" is not a reason that you must be induced or have a cesarean unless you decide you want one. It is best to let labor begin spontaneously and allow it progress naturally. During labor, you should try positions that will help the baby to descend and rotate. Squatting, kneeling, and rocking the pelvis may be helpful. If your labor stalls significantly or if you are unable to push the baby out, then a cesarean may be in order.

Oligohydramnios (Low Amniotic Fluid)

Oligohydramnios is a condition in which the amount of amniotic fluid around the baby is low. One liter of fluid is produced every day from the baby's urine and lung secretions. The baby then swallows the fluid and turns it into urine again. If the placenta is old (the pregnancy has passed the due date) or not working well, the fetus doesn't receive adequate oxygen and its urine production declines. Therefore, the measurement of amniotic fluid is touted as an indirect test of fetal health. The amniotic fluid also acts as a cushion within the uterus to give the baby room to move and grow.

Low levels of fluid are found in 5 percent of pregnancies but may be as high as 11 percent in women who have passed their due date. Fluid levels peak at thirty-four weeks and then naturally decline as the pregnancy nears the due date.

To determine the amount of fluid around the baby, a doctor will measure it with an ultrasound. An accurate measurement of the fluid depends on the skill of the ultrasound technician and the position of the baby. Fluid pockets located between the baby and the mother's spine cannot be measured precisely. Often, oligohydramnios is found incidentally on an ultrasound that is being done to confirm the baby's position or size.

Oligohydramnios is associated with an increased risk of medical interventions, such as multiple ultrasounds, fetal monitoring, and labor induction. However, researchers now believe that low fluid alone is not a good indicator of fetal well-being. In a commonly used obstetrical textbook, an expert in the field admits that "investigators have tried, with mixed success, to demonstrate the utility and applicability of ultrasound examination of amniotic fluid volume (AFV) in relation to perinatal outcome. Despite overwhelming evidence that any ultrasound methods for predicting AFV is poor at best, clinical practice continues to include it."[7] Translation: Measuring the amniotic fluid doesn't tell us whether your baby is healthy, but we still do it all the time. If low fluid is the only abnormal finding, outcomes for the baby are similar to pregnancies with normal fluid. Yet, a survey of OBs in 2009 showed that 91 percent still believe that low fluid was associated with poor outcomes and that labor should be induced in cases of oligohydramnios.

If your doctor recommends labor induction because of low fluid, you should clarify whether there are other concerns about your baby as well. Are there any birth defects? Is the baby moving well? Is the size of the baby normal? How is your blood pressure? If no other problems are identified, you can ask your provider whether you can drink fluids and then be retested. Maternal hydration, IV or oral, increases amniotic fluid volume significantly. Drinking 2 liters of water over two hours can raise it by 60 percent.

If the fluid is still low and your doctor insists on induction, you can politely tell him that you have done some research on the subject and would like to know whether waiting is an option. You can seek a second opinion from another doctor as well. Ultimately, it is your decision whether you are induced.

Placenta Previa

A placenta previa is one that covers the cervix. The placenta adheres to the wall of the uterus and supplies oxygen and nutrition to the growing baby. Normally, the placenta attaches to the side or top of the uterus. In the second trimester, 5 percent of placentas are found at the bottom, covering the cervix. As the uterus grows, the lower part, called the lower uterine segment, expands and the placenta is pulled toward the top. Over 90 percent of placenta previas identified in the second trimester will move spontaneously with only 4 in 1,000 remaining in this position at the due date.

If your doctor tells you that you have a placenta previa when you have your twenty-week ultrasound, do not be alarmed. In the vast majority of cases, the placenta will move out of the way. If you have a previa, you should refrain from intercourse or inserting anything in your vagina, as that could cause the placenta to bleed. Over half of women with a previa in the third trimester will bleed spontaneously, and over one third will require an emergency cesarean.

A vaginal delivery is not possible with a placenta previa. As the cervix opens in early labor, the placenta stretches. Because it contains hundreds of blood vessels, the blood loss can be rapid and can cause death of the fetus within minutes. If your placenta is "low-lying," with the edge of the placenta more than 2 cm away from the cervix, a vaginal delivery may be attempted as long as it is done in a hospital. If there is excessive bleeding, an emergency cesarean can be done.

Women older than forty and smokers are at greatest risk of developing a placenta previa. In addition, if you have previously had a cesarean, the chance of a previa nearly triples. After two cesareans, it increases sevenfold.

For women who were planning a natural, unmedicated birth, the diagnosis of placenta previa can be devastating. There is nothing you can do to make your placenta move. It is best to accept the diagnosis, be grateful for modern medicine—without it, your baby could die during delivery—and find a way to make the unexpected cesarean into a positive experience.

Postterm Pregnancy

A postterm pregnancy is one that lasts more than forty-two weeks. Accurately calculating the due date in early pregnancy is essential to determining which pregnancies are postterm.

Pregnant women love to find out their due date. They want to prepare for the birth, go on a vacation, schedule time off work, arrange care for another child, or make plans for out-of-town family members to be present. When the due date comes and goes, they begin to wonder whether something is wrong, or if the pregnancy will ever end.

Due dates certainly are helpful for monitoring general milestones in the pregnancy that are based on gestational age. For example, we expect that a woman will feel her baby moving by week twenty.

Measuring the fundal height and knowing the gestational age help doctors see whether the baby is growing normally. However, due dates are far from predictive of when a baby will be born. In fact, only 4 percent arrive on their due date, and 50 percent of women will go past the due date. The most common time to deliver is between forty and forty-one weeks, when 31 percent of babies are born.

A baby's organs are fully developed by thirty-nine to forty weeks. The baby is not "more" physically ready if it stays inside longer. But the last few weeks of pregnancy are a critical time for the baby to properly position itself for labor. While it is physically mature, it may not rotate into the correct position for childbirth until after the due date has past.

Many doctors, patients, and their families think of the due date as an absolute deadline. If you share your date, you will have endless calls from friends and family to see whether the baby has come yet. Their well-meaning inquiries translate into pressure to get the baby delivered, or worries about whether it is safe for the baby to stay inside longer. Doctors use the due date as a guide for when they will induce labor.

To establish due dates, doctors use Naegele's rule from 1806: starting with the date of the last menstrual period (LMP), add one year, subtract three months, and add seven days. Naegele's rule was based on the belief that gestation is ten menstrual cycles in duration. More recent studies have debated how accurately Naegele's rule calculates the exact duration of human pregnancy.

We know that ovulation and conception usually occur two weeks after the period starts. Based on Naegele's rule, the length of gestation is 280 days from the first day of the period. However, when we look at pregnancies with spontaneous labor, the average time from the last period to delivery in women having their first baby is 288 days—eight days longer than Naegele's rule suggests.

How long a pregnancy lasts varies considerably. For women whose exact conception date was known, the delivery dates were spread over a thirty-seven-day window. This means that even when we know the date of conception precisely, we cannot predict the exact date of birth, as there is natural variation in the length of human pregnancy.[8]

An ultrasound in the first trimester confirms a baby's gestational age and an approximate due date. The fetal size is measured by determining the distance in millimeters between the crown (head) and rump (buttocks), called the crown-rump length (CRL). There is a specific correlation of the CRL with gestational age. For example, if the CRL is 3.5 mm, the fetus is six weeks. If the CRL is 4.0 mm, the fetus is six weeks one day. In early pregnancy, very small changes in the CRL affect the gestational age estimation. Therefore, the earlier the ultrasound is done, the more accurate it is in determining gestational age and due date. Ultrasounds in the second or third trimester are not as accurate so once a due date is established, it will not be changed. However, while this test accurately determines gestational age, it will not tell us when the pregnancy will end.

Factors influencing when a woman will deliver include:

- How long it took the embryo to implant in the uterus: Embryos that take longer to attach to the uterus have a longer gestation.
- Obesity: Because fat cells store hormones, the hormonal trigger for labor is altered in obese women.
- Family history: If your sister delivered a baby late, you have a 1.8 times risk of being late as well.
- Your personal birth history: If you were born postterm, it is more likely that your baby will follow suit.
- Education: If you are well educated, you have a greater likelihood of being late than uneducated women.
- The sex of the fetus: Male babies are more often late.
- Severe stress: Sudden or extreme stress, such a death in the family, experienced in weeks 33 to 36 of the pregnancy, can prolong the pregnancy.

- Personal history: If a previous pregnancy was late, it is likely that you will deliver late again.
- If you are having your first child: First babies are more likely to arrive late.

Risks Associated with Having a Postterm Pregnancy

- Macrosomia: Excessive birth weight (greater than 4,500 grams [9 pounds 15 ounces]), is found in 5 percent of postterm babies. After the due date, a baby gains 4 to 5 ounces per week.
- Stillbirth: Although the risk clearly increases with length of gestation, the absolute risk is quite low:
  - *40 weeks:* 0.42 per 1,000
  - *41 weeks:* 0.61 per 1,000
  - *42 weeks:* 1.08 per 1,000
  - *43 weeks and above:* 1.58 to 8.5 per 1,000.
- Meconium aspiration syndrome: A fetus is more likely to pass meconium after the due date because its intestinal tract is mature. If a baby breathes in meconium during pregnancy or birth, its lungs may be damaged, known as meconium aspiration syndrome (see page 263).

How Long Is It Safe to Wait?

In a recent survey, 44 percent of women said that their provider suggested labor induction because they were "close to their due date."[9] It has become common practice in the United States to induce labor near forty weeks.

ACOG recommends induction between forty-two and forty-three weeks for uncomplicated pregnancies. Antepartum testing with non-stress tests and exams of the amniotic fluid are routinely started if a woman goes past her due date. However, the studies on the use of antepartum testing prior to forty-two weeks do not show a benefit.

One of the most common reasons that your baby hasn't come out yet is that it isn't in the proper position. You can encourage the baby to drop into the pelvis by staying active, going on walks, and stretching your hips and groin. Your doctor or midwife can also "strip your membranes." This procedure involves using the fingers to separate the amniotic sac from the uterine wall and has been shown to increase the chance of delivering before forty-one weeks. For more about membrane stripping, see page 232. If you have passed your due date and want a natural birth, you can wait until at least forty-two weeks. If your baby is moving well and has a normal heart rate, you may postpone an induction to forty-three weeks. While ACOG supports this guideline, many physicians are not comfortable waiting this long and will pressure you with statistics about stillbirth. Ultimately, you must weigh the pros and cons for yourself.

Preeclampsia

Preeclampsia is a condition that develops after twenty weeks of pregnancy or in the first six weeks postpartum that is characterized by high blood pressure. The elevated pressure causes kidney dysfunction, with protein spilling into the urine. Swelling, especially in the hands and face, can occur. Eventually, it can lead to seizures and even maternal death. Preeclampsia affects 6 to 8 percent of pregnancies and is responsible for over seventy-six thousand maternal deaths per year around the world. In the United States, the incidence of preeclampsia has increased 25 percent in the last two decades.[10]

Hippocrates first described the symptoms of this disease in 400 BC, when pregnant women were observed having severe headaches and seizures. In 1849, Dr. William Smith believed that toxins in the blood were responsible and the condition became known as toxemia. There were other theories as well: that the uterus was too tight, that anxiety and worry were to blame, and even that unstable weather patterns were a factor. In the late 1800s, women with this condition were given medications to purge the body of toxins. Leeches were applied to suck the blood from their bodies. Finally, in 1896, the invention of a manometer to measure blood pressure led doctors to recognize that preeclampsia is related to high blood pressure.

Even today, the exact cause of preeclampsia is unknown. Recent research is focused on the development of abnormal blood vessels within the placenta. Women who develop preeclampsia overproduce certain placental proteins months before the symptoms of the disease are evident. As a result, arteries throughout the body spasm and leak, leading to the high blood pressure and swelling.

Risk Factors for Preeclampsia

Although we do not know the exact cause of preeclampsia, there are a number of health issues and contributing factors that are related to this condition. These include:

- Chronic high blood pressure
- First baby (3-fold risk)
- Renal disease
- Diabetes
- Lupus
- Greater than age 40 (double the risk)
- Obesity
- Previous pregnancy with preeclampsia (7-fold risk)
- Family history: If your mother had preeclampsia, you have a 30 percent chance of developing it. If your sister had it, you have a 20 percent chance.
- Vitamin D: Women with low vitamin D during the first 26 weeks of pregnancy are 40 percent more likely to develop severe preeclampsia but not mild preeclampsia. However, vitamin D levels are not routinely screened during pregnancy because there aren't yet enough studies to support its testing.

Initially, most women with preeclampsia have no symptoms. Receiving the diagnosis may seem inconceivable to some patients because they feel completely normal. Those hoping for a nonin-terventional birth are suddenly faced with a different path, often involving labor induction, continuous fetal monitoring, and bed rest.

Consistent prenatal care is critical to the early detection of pre-eclampsia. At each prenatal visit, your provider will check your blood pressure, examine your urine for protein, and inquire about swelling. Because the incidence of preeclampsia and other compli-cations increases as you get closer to term, your prenatal visits will be more frequent: monthly during the second trimester, biweekly during the early third trimester, and weekly during the last month. If your blood pressure is persistently greater than 140/90 and you have protein in the urine, the diagnosis is confirmed.

Identifying women who are at risk for developing preeclampsia is an area of active research. Certain markers in the blood, such as placental growth factor (PGF), can be measured to predict this disorder. Almost half of women with low PGF levels will develop preeclampsia in the following two weeks. While these markers are helpful in identifying the risk of preeclampsia, there is little that can be done to prevent it.

The blood pressure pattern during pregnancy can also predict this disease. Normally, blood pressure decreases by ten points during the second trimester, with the lowest readings between six-teen to twenty weeks. Women who do not have this natural drop are more likely to develop preeclampsia.

the doctor's diary

My first pregnancy had been going smoothly. I was thirty-four years old and expecting a boy. I was driving to work one morning at twen-ty-nine weeks and felt a strange fog in my head. I didn't have a head-ache; rather, I felt like I couldn't think straight. I had slept well the night before but was still somewhat groggy. I went through my day, seeing patients, and delivering a baby in the afternoon. All day, this fog hung over me. I was forgetful and drowsy. At the end of the day, I asked one of my nurses to check my blood pressure. I was shocked to see that it was 160/110—the standard is 120/80—but was sure that it was just nerves. My partner in medical practice, also an ob-gyn, sent me to the hospital. Reading after reading showed my blood pressure to be very high.

Over the next two weeks, I rested in bed, wanting to stay pregnant as long as I could. That was all I could do, because there is no treatment. Of course, studies have shown that bed rest doesn't help, and it didn't for me. I kept getting sicker. At that point, my son was only 3 pounds, so I wanted him to stay inside as long as possible. I never had the headaches, blurred vision, or abdominal pain that is common with preeclampsia. However, that foggy feeling was there, every day. At thirty-one weeks, I woke up to find my face, hands, and arms incredibly swollen. My family thought that I looked like the Michelin man. I went to the hospital and blood tests showed I now had HELLP. HELLP is a specific syndrome that results from preeclampsia:

> **H (hemolysis):** Red blood cells break down, causing anemia.
> **EL (elevated liver enzymes):** The liver doesn't work normally.
> **LP (low platelets):** The platelets that are responsible for blood clotting are destroyed.

Now I had no other choice but to be delivered. I was induced and had a vaginal birth. My son weighed 3 pounds, had a bleed in his brain from prematurity, and spent six weeks in the neonatal intensive care unit (NICU). Fortunately, he had no long-term health issues. Now a teenager, he is taller than me and perfect!

Preeclampsia leads to millions of preterm births every year. It also can cause poor fetal growth and stillbirth. The earlier preeclampsia develops, the more likely that it will be severe.

The only cure for preeclampsia is delivery. Medications and bed rest are not effective. Unfortunately, the course of this disease is irreversible as well as unpredictable. Some women have a mild case that persists for months, whereas others have blood pressure readings that rise rapidly over just a few days. The timing of delivery seeks to balance what is best for the mother with what is best for the baby. If the baby is significantly premature, doctors may choose to wait as long as possible. But once the mother's health is in danger, the baby must be delivered.

Having slightly elevated blood pressure is common in the last month of pregnancy. If high blood pressure is the only abnormality, the diagnosis of "gestational hypertension" is made. Women with gestational hypertension may be allowed to wait for spontaneous labor or for signs of preeclampsia.

Preventing Preeclampsia

There are some actions you can take to reduce your risk of getting preeclampsia.

- Modify risk factors: Take action before pregnancy to reduce or eliminate such risk factors as diabetes, high blood pressure, or obesity.
- Take aspirin: If you had preeclampsia in a previous pregnancy, take low-dose ("baby") aspirin. It can reduce the risk of having preeclampsia a second time by 10 to 30 percent. The recommended dosage of aspirin is 81 mg per day, but only if your doctor or midwife agrees.
- Take calcium: Calcium supplements of at least 1,000 mg per day greatly reduced the risk of preeclampsia, but only if your normal daily calcium intake was less than 1,000 mg per day.
- Exercise: Physical activity during early pregnancy increases blood flow and plays a role in placental development. When exercising, levels of placental growth factor are higher, which may protect a mother from preeclampsia.

Approaches that have found to be *ineffective* in preventing preeclampsia include: decreasing salt intake, decreasing activity, garlic, vitamin C, vitamin E, and bed rest.

Preterm Labor (PTL)

Preterm labor is uterine contractions that dilate the cervix prior to thirty-seven weeks of gestation. The incidence of preterm birth in the United States has risen 30 percent since the 1980s, and now accounts for 11 percent of deliveries. Preterm birth is the leading cause of death in children under age five. The United States has one of the highest rates of preterm birth of developed countries.

Contractions prior to the time for delivery are common. The majority of these are Braxton Hicks contractions or "false labor," in which the uterine muscle tightens but only a low level of pressure is produced and the cervix does not dilate. With true labor, the contractions are strong and the pressure is high. You can distinguish Braxton Hicks from true labor by monitoring the intensity and regularity of the contractions. If you feel a tightness but it does not cause you to catch your breath, you most likely are having Braxton Hicks contractions. True contractions are rhythmic, whereas Braxton Hicks are irregular, occurring less than eight times per hour. In addition, with true contractions, you will likely have mucus discharge that may contain blood.

The only way to confirm if you are in preterm labor is a cervical exam. If your cervix is not dilated or effaced, you are not in labor. In addition, a vaginal swab to detect the presence of fetal fibronectin can be done. Fetal fibronectin is a protein that acts as a glue to attach the bag of water to the uterus. As your body prepares to go into labor, this protein breaks down and can be found in the vagina. If your fetal fibronectin test is negative, your chance of delivering in the next two weeks is less than 1 percent and you can be reassured that you are not in preterm labor. If your test is positive, you have a 25 percent chance of delivering soon.

The cause of most cases of preterm labor is unknown. Some are the result of infections, including urinary tract infections, vaginal infections like bacterial vaginosis, and periodontal disease. Others are due to having twins, smoking, having a short cervix, or being excessively stressed. If you have had a previous preterm delivery, you have a 50 percent chance of having another one. If you are carrying twins or are under twenty years old, you are also at an increased risk.

Preventing Preterm Birth

There are some strategies you can adopt to prevent preterm birth.

- Stop smoking.
- Sleep sufficiently: Get 8 hours of sleep each night.
- Reduce stress: There is an increased risk of preterm birth for women diagnosed with anxiety and for those who have experienced a stressful life event, especially during the first trimester.
- Take vitamin D: Vitamin D enhances the immune system's response to infections and suppresses inflammation. Both of these mechanisms may help to prevent preterm birth.
- Maintain good nutrition: Women eating a balanced diet, including fruits, vegetables, and fish, can decrease their risk of preterm birth by 15 percent.
- Eat fish: One study showed that the risk of preterm birth was reduced by 13 percent in women who eat fish at least 3 times per week.[11]
- Increase omega-3: Omega-3 fatty acid supplements may also be helpful.
- Maintain a healthy vaginal flora: *Lactobacillus acidophilus* is the most common organism in the vaginal canal. When lactobacillus levels decline, other bacteria thrive, a condition known as bacterial vaginosis (BV). BV increases the risk of preterm labor by 40 percent. Replenishing lactobacillus with probiotics (10^9 to 10^{11} colony-forming units (CFU) daily) can help to prevent BV.
- If you are trying to get pregnant using IVF: decrease the risk of twins and triplets by having your fertility doctor transfer a single embryo into the uterus.

- Postpone elective delivery: Do not schedule an elective cesareans or labor induction prior to 39 weeks. While this recommendation won't stop preterm labor, it prevents preterm birth. In the past, elective inductions and cesareans were done after 37 weeks—since that is considered "full term." However, babies born electively between 37 and 39 weeks may have respiratory issues and are admitted to the NICU more frequently. Therefore, elective deliveries should only be scheduled at 39 weeks or later.

Although many medications have been tried, none has been proven to prolong pregnancy for more than a few days. The following treatments for preterm labor are also *not* effective: vitamin C, magnesium, calcium, hydration, abstaining from sex, and bed rest.

Multiple studies prove that bed rest does not prevent preterm birth. Yet, doctors continue to prescribe it regularly, largely because no other treatments are available. While the idea of lying down and resting seems a logical approach, it has never been proven to work. In fact, the stress associated with bed rest actually causes women to deliver earlier.

If you are truly in preterm labor, your doctor will give you steroids to help your baby's lungs develop more quickly and to protect against bleeding in the baby's brain after delivery. Steroids reduce the risk of a baby's dying from complications of prematurity by nearly 40 percent. They are most effective when given at least 48 hours before delivery. Therefore, you may be given medication to stop your contractions temporarily so that the steroids have time to take effect. There are no risks, and only benefits, to you or the baby from using steroids.

If you have previously delivered a baby early, you may be a candidate for progestin therapy. The hormone 17-hydroxyprogesterone caproate (17OH-PC) reduces the chance of recurrent preterm birth by one third. Known by its trade name Makena, it is given as a weekly injection beginning at sixteen weeks. Any woman with a history of a delivery prior to thirty-five weeks is encouraged to take this medication with her next pregnancy.

Short Cervix

Shaped like a cylinder and 3 to 5 cm in length, the cervix is the lowest part of the uterus that extends into the vagina. During pregnancy, it fills with a thick mucus that protects the fetus from infections. During childbirth, it opens to allow the baby to pass through.

If your cervix shortens too early, it may not be able to hold the baby in until the due date, resulting in a preterm birth. A woman with a short cervix has a sixfold increased risk of delivering prematurely. A cervix may be short as the result of a prior surgery, such as a treatment for an abnormal Pap smear, cervical insufficiency in which the cervical tissue is naturally weak, an infection, or a drop in progesterone levels.

Occurring in 10 percent of pregnancies, a "short" cervix measures fewer than 25 millimeters in the second trimester. The shorter the cervix, the greater the risk for preterm birth.

Cervical length	Average time of delivery
10 mm	32 weeks
10–15 mm	33 weeks
15–20 mm	34 weeks

Women with a history of preterm birth should be screened with a vaginal ultrasound in the second trimester to check for cervical shortening. Some doctors will routinely screen all their patients, even if they haven't had a preterm birth, because the consequences of preterm birth are so significant.

Treatments for a Short Cervix

Depending on the length of the cervix, as well as a number of other considerations, your doctor will give you some options to try to avoid preterm birth. Most women with a short cervix can have a vaginal delivery.

If your cervix is found to be short and you do not have a history of preterm birth, you may be given a daily vaginal suppository of progesterone. While there are no medications to stop preterm labor, this medicine has been shown to prolong pregnancy in women with a short cervix.

If you have a short cervix as well as a history of preterm delivery, the approach is multifaceted. Your doctor may offer you a cervical cerclage in addition to vaginal progesterone suppositories and weekly progestin injections. A cervical cerclage is a stitch that your ob-gyn will place in the cervix to hold it closed.

Another treatment for a short cervix is a cervical pessary. A pessary is a rubber ring-shaped device that is placed in the vagina. By pushing on the walls of the vagina, the pessary shifts the weight of the uterus away from the cervix. Cervical pessaries are not available in the United States because they are not FDA-approved. Some international studies have shown positive outcomes with this device without significant side effects. More studies are needed to prove if it is an effective and inexpensive way to prolong pregnancy.

Forty percent of women with a short cervix are prescribed "activity restriction."[12] They are told by their doctor to abstain from sex, stop working, and remain on bed rest. However, women who restrict their activity are actually 2.5 times *more likely* to deliver preterm than are women without restrictions. Instead of preventing preterm birth, anxiety and stress from being at bed rest actually makes it more likely.

Threatened Abortion and Miscarriage

Seeing those two blue lines on the pregnancy test inspires you to think about the future of your family with this new life in it. A mom can't help but wonder whether it'll be a boy or girl, what he will look like, whose nose he'll have. The bonding begins immediately. Whether a few weeks into the pregnancy or a few months, any sign of bleeding causes women to fear the worst—am I having a miscarriage?

A threatened abortion is vaginal bleeding that occurs during the first half of pregnancy (prior to twenty weeks). Nearly 30 percent of women experience this type of bleeding. Of those, half will go on to have a miscarriage. Most miscarriages occur very early, before a fetal heartbeat is seen on the ultrasound. Once the heartbeat is seen, around six weeks, the chance of having a miscarriage drops to 5 percent.

If you have bleeding, your provider will check for any other sources of the blood, such as a cervical polyp, or vaginal infection, such as bacterial vaginosis, yeast, chlamydia, or trichomonas. An ultrasound will be done to determine the health of the pregnancy, checking for the presence of the amniotic sac, the fetus, and its heartbeat. If bleeding occurs in the second trimester, an ultrasound of the cervix may also be done to determine if it is short. If the vaginal bleeding is heavy or extends into the second trimester, the risk for preterm birth increases threefold.

The most common cause of a threatened abortion when the pregnancy is otherwise healthy is a blood clot that forms between the amniotic sac and the wall of the uterus, called a subchorionic hematoma. When the pregnancy attaches to the uterine wall, hundreds of delicate new blood vessels are formed. Sometimes, these vessels break and bleed, causing the blood to accumulate between the sac and the uterus. Eventually, the blood is reabsorbed into the body, but some of it makes its way out through the vagina. The majority of subchorionic hematomas do not affect the pregnancy in any way. However, the vaginal bleeding may last for a few weeks. You do not need to restrict your activities; the hematoma will resolve on its own.

The idea of miscarriage is still shrouded in misinformation and guilt. A recent national survey found that the majority of people, especially men, believe that miscarriage occurs infrequently—less than 5 percent of pregnancies.[13] Miscarriage is actually the most common pregnancy complication, occurring in 20 percent of pregnancies, and is even more common in older women. At age forty, the risk of having a pregnancy loss is 1 in 3.

In addition, many people still believe that miscarriage is caused by things that a woman can control: lifting heavy items, using birth control pills, having an STD, or getting in an argument. However, none of these actually triggers miscarriage. Instead, the majority of pregnancy losses, nearly 80 percent, are caused by genetic abnormalities in the fetus. To take two cells, one from a mother and one from a father, combine them, and then have them grow and divide into thousands is truly astounding. For a fetus to grow normally, the cells must divide correctly and the chromosomes must split perfectly. The fact that this process occurs without mistakes as often as it does is impressive. In cases of genetic abnormalities, a miscarriage is the body's natural way of letting go of a pregnancy that would not have been healthy. Most pregnancies are lost in the early first trimester, prior to the development of a fetal heartbeat.

Other Common Causes of Miscarriage
- Malformations of the uterus
- Autoimmune diseases, such as lupus
- Untreated medical problems, such as diabetes or thyroid disease

Most miscarriages are not preventable. If you have bleeding in early pregnancy and the fetus is healthy, the bleeding will likely resolve. If your bleeding is associated with a pregnancy with a genetic abnormality, you will miscarry no matter what you do. Doctors have suggested the use of vitamins, Chinese herbs, medicine to stop uterine contractions, and pregnancy hormone supplements, to no avail. Neither do bed rest, limiting excessive activity, and refraining from sex improve outcomes. The use of the hormone progesterone to prevent miscarriage is controversial. While it is not beneficial to take progesterone if you are bleeding, it may decrease the chance of miscarriage for women with at least two previous miscarriages.

the doctor's diary

When I have to tell a new mom that her pregnancy isn't growing normally, I am saddened as well. I will search the ultrasound screen for minutes, looking for any sign of a heartbeat. But the truth is that I know immediately when I see the picture. A strong heartbeat jumps off the screen. When I don't see it, I bide my time by looking around longer, trying to craft the right way to deliver the bad news. There are no easy words. Some moms are in disbelief; others had an intimation—maybe they didn't feel pregnant, or had some bleeding. No matter what, the reality is devastating.

Twins

Twins comprise just over 3 percent of all births in the United States. Of those, one third are conceived naturally and two thirds are the result of fertility treatments. Between 1980 and 2010, the twinning rate has increased 76 percent.

A twin pregnancy is always exciting but carries with it unique risks, since two babies are sharing a space ideally designed for one. Preeclampsia, preterm labor, hyperemesis, and gestational diabetes all occur more frequently in women carrying twins. The average time to deliver twins is thirty-six weeks of gestation. They are usually smaller than singletons, weighing 5 pounds each.

Many women carrying twins are automatically prescribed bed rest for most of the pregnancy. However, bed rest does not prevent the preterm delivery of twins, even for women who are having contractions. In fact, women who stay in bed are more likely to deliver early compared to those who continue their normal activities.

How Should Twins Be Delivered?

At least 75 percent of twin pregnancies in the United States are delivered by scheduled cesarean. Research from the 1980s and 1990s showed a lower complication rate for twins delivered surgically, so this became the accepted norm. Many physicians today will not give their patients with twins the option to deliver vaginally.

Vaginal delivery of twins is considered "risky" because of what happens *after* the first baby is born. Delivery of the first baby, if it is head down, is essentially the same as a singleton birth. However, after twin A is born, twin B suddenly has extra room within the uterus. The twin can spin around and move side to side, as it never could during the pregnancy. It can become entangled in its umbilical cord or may try to come out sideways, instead of head or feet first. If the second twin settles into a head-down position, it can be delivered vaginally, with the forces of the uterine contractions and the mother's pushing efforts. However, if twin B ends up breech or sideways, a skilled provider, who is trained in internal podalic version, can reach his hand though the dilated cervix and into the uterus, grabbing both feet of twin B and guiding the baby through the birth canal. These deliveries are ideally done in a hospital, with a second physician using the ultrasound to monitor twin B. If twin B cannot be delivered safely vaginally, a cesarean will be done for this baby. The mother will end up with a vaginal delivery and a cesarean on the same day!

To determine whether you are a good candidate for vaginal delivery of twins, your provider will consider the gestational age, the size, and the positions of your babies. If you are thirty-two weeks or greater and twin A is head down, a vaginal birth is as safe as a planned cesarean.[14]

Most doctors will only attempt a vaginal delivery of twins if the first twin is head down, to avoid the additional risks that are associated with breech delivery, such as head entrapment. In addition, if the first twin is breech and the second is vertex, the chins of the two can become locked together. While this scenario is extremely rare, almost one-third of locked twins will die during delivery.

Most providers consider twins to be a high-risk delivery that should be done in a hospital with skilled physicians on hand. But because many doctors won't offer a vaginal birth to their patients with twins, some moms can't find a doctor to support their wishes and choose a midwife to deliver their twins at home. Some states that regulate midwives, such as California, have laws that forbid twin deliveries in the home. Without any options for a physician to assist in a vaginal delivery, some people do it anyway.

When your plans change for the sake of your health or the health of your baby, you may need to adjust your expectations about having a natural birth. Working with your provider, and keeping the goal of a healthy you and a healthy baby firmly in mind, you can have a positive birth experience no matter what comes your way.

WHAT YOU NEED TO KNOW, AND NEED TO ASK, ABOUT LABOR

If you've decided that a natural birth is your goal, and you don't have time to read everything in this chapter, here's the shorthand version of how to succeed:

Don't go to the hospital immediately when your labor starts. Wait until you are in active labor, when your contractions are painful enough that you can't talk through them or you are having bloody show (discharge that is pink or brown with blood).

Make your delivery area comfortable. Hospitals are full of noises, bright lights, and unfamiliar equipment. You can bring things from home, such as blankets, pillows, pictures, and music, to make the birthing room more personal.

Move around during labor. Try different positions and let your body guide you to a comfortable place.

Have multiple plans for pain management and don't hold on to any one of them too tightly. You can't just wing it! Try deep breathing. If that doesn't work, get in the shower or tub. If that doesn't work, use visualization. The more options you have, the better. Practice these approaches to pain management during pregnancy.

Don't crowd your delivery room with people who are going to watch you every minute. Make your room quiet, peaceful, and private while having a few support people who can reassure and comfort you.

When, and How, Am I Going to Have This Baby?

What triggers labor is still a complex mystery to scientists. The timing is determined by the maturity of the fetus as well as the physical readiness of the mother. Long ago, physicians believed that the baby kicked its way out of its mother by pushing against the top of the uterus with its feet. Despite one hundred years of modern obstetrics and the evolution of our understanding of the hormonal signals between mother and baby, we cannot pinpoint exactly what starts the process.

Your body begins to prepare for labor four to six weeks prior to your first real contraction. During most of pregnancy, the cervix is firm and feels like the tip of a nose. As the due date nears, it becomes softer, like a sponge. Hormonelike substances called prostaglandins cause the cervix to soften, or ripen, as well as to shorten, or efface, going from its original 3 to 5 cm in length to the thinness of a piece of paper.

While these changes can be imperceptible, there are some noticeable signs that the body is getting ready for the big day. As the cervix thins, it releases the mucus plug, a jellylike substance that prevents vaginal bacteria from entering the uterus. The mucus plug may come out as a solid blob or appear as an increase in vaginal discharge over a few weeks. Your discharge may be thick or watery, clear or blood-tinged. The loss of the mucus plug can happen anytime from a month before labor to the day of active labor, and it means that the labor process has begun.

Some patients take a picture of their mucus plug and send it to me, asking what it is. Others have collected it in a tissue or a plastic food storage container and brought it to my office. As much as I appreciate that they want to know exactly what is going on, a verbal description is just fine!

Engagement of the fetal head, or lightening, occurs next. As the lower part of the uterus (the lower uterine segment) thins and stretches, the fetus moves into the pelvis. You will notice more space between your ribs and the baby, making your breathing easier. You may also feel pressure in your lower abdomen and back and the need to urinate often. Bowel movements become soft and more frequent, also as a result of prostaglandins. Braxton Hicks contractions (see page 174) are common and the baby may seem to move less as it runs out of space.

The first eight months of pregnancy is dominated by a state of uterine "quiescence," in which uterine contractions are suppressed by the hormones progesterone, relaxin, and prostacyclin. Around thirty-five weeks, these hormones release their control, and the uterus is "activated." The fetus is also involved in the activation of the uterus by producing a special form of estrogen. When the time for delivery has arrived, prostaglandins and oxytocin stimulate the uterus to contract. The transition from quiescence to activation occurs over the course of days to weeks.

The Natural Progress of Labor

Labor is the process by which regular contractions of the uterus cause the cervix to open and the fetus to move through the birth canal. Labor lasts from a few hours to a few days. While uterine contractions are a significant part of the process, a successful vaginal delivery also depends on the ability of the cervix to soften and the fetus to navigate through the pelvis.

The stages of labor were first described by Dr. Emanuel Friedman in the 1950s. Dr. Friedman identified common patterns of labor by evaluating five hundred first-time mothers. Although these data were collected over sixty years ago, the Friedman curve—which plots cervical dilation versus time on a graph—is still used regularly to identify abnormal labors.

Friedman described three distinct stages of labor:

The first stage: The first stage of labor is the time in which uterine contractions are causing cervical dilation. The cervix must dilate to 10 cm so as to accommodate the 10 cm fetal head. The first stage is divided into two phases: the latent phase and the active phase. The latent phase, which can last a day or two, begins when you first perceive contractions as the cervix opens from zero to 6 cm. In the beginning, you may be unsure whether this is the "real thing." For some women, contractions in this phase are irregular, last thirty to forty-five seconds, and feel like a tightening with a low level of pain, allowing them to rest, nap, and eat. Other women find the contractions of the latent phase very painful right from the beginning.

In the active phase of the first stage, the cervix dilates from 6 to 10 cm, about 1 cm per hour. Active phase contractions occur every two to three minutes, are very painful, and last one minute each. You cannot carry on a conversation during a contraction because of its intensity. Your thought process becomes instinctive and focused. You may alternate between deep breathing and moaning with the contraction and resting and rejuvenating during the minutes in between.

While it is not recognized as a separate phase of labor, many providers will use the term *transition* to describe the last part of the active phase when contractions are most intense and occur every one to two minutes. Transition only lasts for about an hour, but it is the time when you are most likely to lose your focus, request pain medication, or shake uncontrollably. You may not be able to find a comfortable position and have difficulty catching your breath.

The second stage of labor begins at full cervical dilation. The fetus descends through the birth canal with the force of the uterine contractions and the maternal effort of pushing, and is born.

The third stage of labor is the delivery of the placenta.

While Friedman's data is still used regularly by providers to identify abnormalities in labor patterns, many things have changed since the 1950s that influence the rate of labor:

- Epidurals: Much more common today, epidurals add 1 to 2 hours to the second stage.
- Obesity: The obesity rates have doubled in the last 50 years. A thick layer of fat on the abdomen and within the walls of the birth canal create resistance to the baby's coming out, leading to a cesarean rate above 50 percent in obese women.
- Older maternal age: The average age of a first-time mother has increased from 20 to 26.
- Being confined to bed: Continuous fetal monitoring has forced many women to stay in bed during labor.
- Forceps: Over half of the patients in the 1950s were delivered using forceps, significantly shortening the length of the second stage.

Today, the duration of labor is much longer than it was sixty years ago. The active phase is significantly slower than the rate suggested by Friedman. In addition, many patients go long periods of time without any dilation at all, and then resume normal progress, a pattern Friedman didn't record or address. What Friedman's curve defined as the lowest acceptable rate of progress is actually the average for women giving birth today. While many doctors are aware of the more recent and accurate data on the length of labor, the Friedman curve is still commonly referenced.

the doctor's diary

The biggest problem with the Friedman curve is that many doctors adhere to it strictly, even though recent data suggest that it isn't accurate for women today. Many patients have received Pitocin or had cesareans because their labor didn't follow the Friedman curve. Midwives tend to be more flexible with these guidelines and tolerate babies taking their time. Thankfully, new residents in training are now being taught to be patient with labor and allow time to pass as well.

When to Go to the Hospital or Birthing Center

If you are a first-time mom, you may not know if you are in labor because you have nothing to compare it to. Arriving at the hospital too early greatly increases your chance of medical interventions, such as having an IV, continuous fetal monitoring, an epidural, and a cesarean. Nurses, doctors, and even you and your family may become impatient with a long latent phase. Protocols vary from hospital to hospital, but most will admit you if you are at least 4 cm dilated.

You should arrive at your hospital or birthing center when your contractions have been three to five minutes apart for at least a few hours. They should last for sixty seconds each and be strong enough that you cannot carry on a conversation.

the doctor's diary

Some moms request to stay in the hospital even if they aren't in active labor because they are nervous about what is coming next and afraid that labor may get out of hand at home. Latent labor can be long and exhausting. You should try to rest as much as possible at home during this early phase, to avoid unnecessary interventions.

If you are having a home birth, your midwife will give you instructions on when to call her. Most midwives would like to know whether your water has broken or you have started contracting. Once your contractions are regular and strong, your midwife will arrive at your house.

Cervical Exams

When you arrive on the labor and delivery unit, a doctor, midwife, or nurse will perform a cervical exam to determine how dilated you are. The exam also confirms that the baby is in the head-down position and whether your water has broken.

Cervical exams are subjective and can vary among different providers. One nurse may say you are 6 cm; later, a different nurse may say you are 4 cm, giving the impression that the dilation is going backward.

Similar to cervical exams during pregnancy, the cervical exam during labor assesses how much progress has been made, but will not tell you when you will deliver. In fact, for some women, predictions of the birth time are off-putting, making them feel as if they are "on the clock" and not doing something right if they don't deliver "on time." Frequent exams can erode your confidence. If you hear that the cervical exam hasn't changed, you may feel discouraged. Additionally, with each exam the chance of introducing bacteria into the uterus, causing newborn infection, rises. On average, a woman receives seven exams during labor.

If you are showing signs of being in active labor, you don't need frequent cervical exams, or, frankly, any at all. You will instinctively know when to push because you will feel a different sensation, like a pressure on the rectum, as if you need to have a bowel movement.

I think an initial cervical exam is important to confirm that active labor has begun and that the baby's head is down. If you already had an ultrasound or a cervical exam in the last month that confirmed the baby's position, this initial exam can be waived. Having numerous exams during routine labor isn't helpful. With each exam, you must interrupt the rhythm of your breathing to lie down in the bed while the doctor or nurse performs this uncomfortable procedure. Many patients will have two or more different people performing these exams during labor, with differing results, which can add to confusion or frustration. You can let your provider and nurse know that you would like to minimize cervical exams unless they are truly necessary.

How Do You Know Whether Your Water Has Broken?

The amniotic sac encloses the fetus, placenta, and the amniotic fluid within the uterus. It is made of two clear, thin membranes—the amnion and the chorion. The amniotic fluid gives the baby space to move and grow and the sac protects it from bacteria in the vaginal canal. The proteins collagen and fibronectin form the sac's strong matrix. As your due date approaches, enzymes weaken this matrix. In addition to the enzyme's effect, contractions stretch the uterus and pull on the membranes, causing them to break. Although it can happen at any time, if left to nature, most amniotic sacs will break around the time that the cervix is completely dilated.

Distinguishing among the water breaking, the release of the mucus plug, leakage of urine, and the increased vaginal discharge of late pregnancy can be challenging. When the water breaks, you may feel a sudden gush of warm fluid or even a "pop." Amniotic fluid is normally clear but may be slightly pink or yellow. A handy test to see whether your water has broken is to put on a maxi pad and walk around. If the pad is soaked after an hour, it is likely that it is amniotic fluid.

To confirm whether your water broke, your provider can collect the fluid with a vaginal swab. In a test called Amni-Sure, the fluid is analyzed for the presence of a protein (placental alpha-microglobulin) that is only found in high levels in amniotic fluid. The test is over 99 percent accurate and results are available in a few minutes.

The Hormones of Labor

Hormones have a significant role during labor. Estrogen, produced by the placenta, prepares the uterine muscle to contract. Prostaglandins made within the uterus itself are responsible for cervical ripening. The brain's beta-endorphins are natural opioids that relieve pain and stress and assist with postpartum bonding.

Oxytocin produced in the brain is responsible for stimulating uterine contractions during labor as well as releasing milk during breastfeeding. Natural oxytocin has effects on the brain itself, causing a sensation of well-being, calm, and connection. In labor, oxytocin gradually increases, peaking after delivery to cause the uterus to contract firmly to control postpartum bleeding.

Man-made oxytocin, called Pitocin, is used to induce labor as well as make contractions stronger and more frequent. While it has the same chemical structure as oxytocin, it is administered through an IV and cannot pass into the brain, so it does not have the same bonding effects as the natural substance.

The Cardinal Movements of Labor

The cardinal movements of labor are the changes in position of the baby's head that allow it to navigate through its mother's pelvis. There are seven movements seen in every birth:

- Engagement: The head enters the pelvis sideways, in the transverse position, with the eyes facing one of the mother's hips.

- Descent: The head moves lower into the pelvis as its bones overlap, also known as molding.
- Flexion: The fetus flexes its chin so that the diameter of the head is the narrowest.
- Internal rotation: Because a mother's pelvis is wider from front to back than it is from side to side, the head, which is also larger from front to back, must rotate from the transverse position to one in which the back of the baby's head is in the front, near the mother's pubic bone, known as occiput anterior. If the head instead rotates the opposite direction, the back of the head will be near the mother's spine—called occiput posterior.
- Extension: Where the birth canal curves upward, the head and neck extend so the back of head slips under the pubic bone and the head passes out of the vagina.
- External rotation: The baby turns slightly to one side or the other so that its shoulders can fit under the pubic bone. If the baby can't rotate, it can become stuck—the condition called shoulder dystocia (see page 161).
- Expulsion: The rest of the body delivers.

Understanding and Coping with Pain

Pain is integral to the birthing process. It signals that something significant is happening and that you must prepare a safe space to give birth. Without pain, you would be surprised and could give birth in an unprotected setting. Pain also gives cues on how to move and position yourself so that the baby can rotate into the required positions to complete the cardinal movements.

In the first stage of labor, pain comes from the cervix opening, the lower part of the uterus stretching, and the uterine muscle exerting energy. In the second stage of labor, pain results from the uterine muscles contracting as well as the muscles stretching at the opening of the vagina.

The experience of pain during labor is complex and individual. Each woman has different levels of tolerance, ability to cope, and contraction patterns. However, pain must be distinguished from suffering. Suffering is associated with feeling helpless, terrified, out of control, panicked, or distressed. If you are suffering, you need to have your pain relieved.

Not only does pain relief help you, it is also beneficial for your baby. If pain is not addressed and reduced during labor, you can hyperventilate, secrete the stress hormone cortisol, and use excessive oxygen, which decreases the oxygen available to the baby. Uncontrolled pain increases the production of hormones, such as epinephrine, which cause uncoordinated uterine contractions, nausea, fear, and prolonged labor. Anything that reduces pain and supports a mother emotionally will help labor's progress.

the doctor's diary

Most of my patients are afraid of the pain of labor. Some even bring it up at their first prenatal visit. They don't know exactly what to expect but they assume it will be terrible.

Prior to delivery, explore your preconceptions and thoughts about birth. If you view labor as unremittingly painful and scary, you can work on altering that perception. Labor is work, but most women who've gone through it will tell you that giving birth to their baby was one of the most amazing and profound events of their life. There will be a lot more to the experience than pain: excitement, love, an appreciation for the people who are supporting you, and a sense of awe at what your body is capable. Think of the contraction as a force or rush of energy that will propel your baby out. With each surge, you are one step closer to holding your baby.

Women who want to have a natural birth need to prepare pain-relieving techniques in advance. They will, of course, have pain, but they can stay relaxed by utilizing these methods. They can also be assured that if the pain is more than they can handle, standard pain relievers, such as epidurals, are always available. No one should experience birth as suffering.

Natural Pain Relief

Our body is naturally designed to deal with the pain of labor. Endorphins, with their powerful pain-relieving properties, are released from the brain, rise throughout labor, and peak at the time of birth. While endorphins do not eliminate pain completely, they make the process bearable.

Women in labor can achieve pain relief without drugs through a variety of methods. These natural options are more commonly used in a birthing center or at home but can be practiced in a hospital as well.

Acupuncture: A trained practitioner places needles at specific points on the body, called acupuncture sites, which pull energy throughout the body to relieve pain. Women who use acupuncture during labor are less likely to use an epidural.[1]

Birthing ball: A birthing ball is an inflatable rubber ball 2 feet in diameter. By sitting on the ball, a woman applies pressure against her perineum, which reduces the sense of pain.

Breathing: Taking a long, cleansing breath at the end of each contraction relaxes the tension in your muscles. Breathing evenly and slowly through the contraction in early labor and taking shorter shallow breaths during the more intense, active labor can help you to better cope with the pain.

Counterpressure: This technique involves applying pressure to the area of the body where the pain is most intense, such as the lower back. Pressure stimulates large nerve fibers that override the smaller nerve fibers that are transmitting the pain signals.

Heat and cold: Both heat and cold can bring pain relief. Heat can be applied to the back, perineum, or lower abdomen with a heating pad, hot water bottle, or warm compress. Cold can be applied to the face or back through a frozen gel pack, cold water bottle, or cold compress.

Hypnosis: Hypnosis is a state of deep relaxation in which the experience of pain becomes subconscious. Self-hypnosis during labor leads to feeling calm and empowered. Women using this method are less likely to use pain medication.[2]

Intracutaneous injections of sterile water: This technique is rarely used in the United States, but is common in other parts of the world, such as the United Kingdom, Australia, and India. A physician or midwife injects a small amount of sterile water with a thin needle into the skin at four locations on the lower back. The water injections utilize the "gate control" theory of pain, which says that a less painful input closes the gate to a more painful one. This is why we instinctively rub where we've been slapped or when we stub our toe. The rubbing sensation blocks the painful input from the slap or stub. In this case, the small amount of burning pain from the water injection blocks the sensation of deep pain from the uterus. The effect lasts forty-five minutes to two hours.

In one study, over 90 percent of women using this method described a decrease in the intensity and unpleasantness of their contractions.[3]

Massage: Studies prove that massage of the lower back, feet, shoulders, and scalp gave significant emotional and physical relief during labor.[4]

Movement: Women in labor will move instinctively to find a comfortable position. In doing so, they rock their pelvis, which encourages the baby to proceed through its cardinal movements. Women who remain upright during labor use less pain medication, have shorter labors, and have less need for Pitocin. Other movements that can be beneficial include: sitting on a birthing ball or rocking in a chair, squatting, lying on one's side, standing, walking, leaning against a wall for support, and rocking from side to side

You should have space to walk around or a chair to sit in so you are not lying on your back for the duration of labor. If you have continuous fetal monitoring, an IV, or have used pain medication, your movements may be limited.

Music: Music or white noise can be used as a distraction from pain. You can prepare a playlist and listen to it during pregnancy. Then, during labor, the music may be used as a cue to relax, breathe rhythmically, or to elevate your mood.

Rebozos: A rebozo is a 4-foot long piece of fabric that can be used to wrap your belly and back during labor. You can place the cloth under your abdomen. The ends are held by your partner behind you. As you lean forward against a wall or birthing ball, the rebozo lifts your uterus and shifts your weight, straightening your baby's path through the pelvis.

TENS: A portable transcutaneous electrical nerve stimulation (TENS) machine has four electrodes that are placed on your back and emit electric pulses of energy. These pulses send signals to the brain that help with pain relief and distract from contractions, without any side effects. TENS works best for early labor. You can adjust the strength and frequency of the pulses. TENS units are available in medical supply stores without a doctor's prescription in many countries and may be ordered online in the United States.

Visualization: As a distraction from pain, you can use mental images of a restful scene. You should sharpen your skills during pregnancy by figuring out what images you want to focus on and practice using them regularly.

VISUALIZATION

Visualization is important during pregnancy and a great tool during labor. It can be used to rehearse your birth in your mind and picture your perfect birth. What will the room look like? Which positions are comfortable for you? You can try these suggestions:

- Waves in the Ocean: Imagine that you are on a white sandy beach. You feel the hot sun on your skin and smell the salty air. You wade into warm clear water and float effortlessly in the small ripples. You are buoyant. You get closer to the surf. As each contraction strengthens, you ride to the peak of the wave. As it releases, you come down the other side. The intensity of transition is like the waves crashing. You feel that you won't make it to the shore but you are strong, and you swim through the white wash safely to the sand.
- The Balloon: With each contraction, you picture a balloon filling slowly. The balloon gets larger and larger to the peak of the contraction. It then floats into the sky as the pain decreases.
- Hill Climber: You are climbing up a hill with each contraction. You take long purposeful breaths as you reach the peak of the hill. As the contraction peaks, you relax your body to slowly walk down the other side.

Vocalization: Low, deep sounds, such as low moaning (not screaming), can be very relaxing, focusing, and peaceful.

Water immersion: Many women agree that the idea of a warm bath during labor sounds inviting. The use of water immersion as a relaxation technique has gained popularity. About 6 percent of women in the United States use this method during labor. Midwives encourage water immersion, with 40 percent of their patients using a bath.

Warmth and buoyancy relieve muscular tension and reduce pressure on your back. Being in the water also decreases the release of stress hormones, which enhances the progression of labor, shortening the first stage by thirty minutes. However, prolonged immersion in the tub may actually slow labor by decreasing natural oxytocin production. Therefore, it is best to enter the tub once active labor has begun and to limit the time in the tub to less than two hours at a time. The water in the tub should be maintained at 97 to 99.5 degrees Fahrenheit. You can safely be in the tub even if your water has broken.

Many hospitals now have labor and delivery suites with tubs for water immersion. If the hospital is not equipped with them, a tub can also be rented from a private company and delivered to the hospital. You can ask your provider what is available in your area.

WATER BIRTH

According to ACOG, water birth is experimental and its safety has not been well established. While the benefits of water immersion during the first stage of labor are well documented, very few studies look at delivering the baby underwater. The first study to review the experience of underwater births in the United States was published in the *Journal of Midwifery* in 2016.[5] Over 6,500 mothers gave birth underwater at home and in birthing centers. The newborns had similar outcomes to babies born outside of the water and fewer transfers to a hospital after birth. In addition, there was no increased risk of infection in the mothers.

The benefits of water birth include decreased pain, gentler transition, and less vaginal trauma. For the baby, the potential complications are infection, umbilical cord rupture when the baby is removed from water, respiratory distress, and aspiration of water. While there are no scientific studies to confirm why a baby doesn't try to breathe while underwater, some have postulated that there is a protective "diving reflex." Stress can override this reflex so that the baby may try to breathe while still submerged. Therefore, only babies with a normal heart rate pattern should be born underwater. The doctor or midwife should bring the baby to the surface immediately before the first breath is taken.

I support water births, but have never done one myself because my hospital, like most, doesn't allow them. Anecdotally, women enjoy the experience, feel relaxed in the water, and the recent data suggest that it is safe. I hope that there will be more studies by scientists to look at safety issues and to understand the physiology of what happens to a baby born underwater.

Having Supportive People

Planning for your birth with a group of supportive friends and family is especially helpful if you are planning a natural delivery. You should talk to them ahead of time so they understand your goals and needs. They can bring soothing music, give a massage, help you focus on a relaxing image, or assist you in moving around the room. They can fetch water, snacks, or cold washcloths for your forehead. They can ask questions of the doctor and nurse if you don't understand something.

The people you invite to be with you as you labor should be there to support you, not to tell horror stories of their own births, play on their phones, look at the clock, watch TV, sit in a chair staring at you, or sleep. Choose them carefully! I have seen family members discussing totally unrelated topics, watching reality TV shows, and paying bills as the mother labors, without offering any support. If they are not going to be helpful, they should not be there. You should also avoid inviting people who make you nervous. No one is entitled to be at the birth of a child other than the parents.

Keep in mind that your birth is not a sporting event. Some patients invite over a dozen friends and family members to be with them. If you want to have a natural birth, having a group of spectators watching you will likely not be helpful. You need to have a quiet, private space in which you can fully relax. My recommendation is to keep it small—just your partner and your doula or one other person.

Fathers' Involvement

It has been accepted since the 1970s that a father attends the birth of his child. Now, nearly all dads are in the delivery room. Most families see it as a necessity. But is having dad in the delivery room helpful or harmful?

In 1965, Dr. Robert Bradley published a book called *Husband-Coached Childbirth*, which encouraged dads to get involved. It taught women to manage the pain of labor with the support of their partner. The approach to birth that he put forth in his book is commonly known as the Bradley method (see page 108). Although Bradley classes help fathers learn how to be supportive, most dads haven't taken this intensive, twelve-week course. As a result, they aren't sure how to help.

Overall, there is little guidance for dads-to-be on what they should or shouldn't do during labor. Theoretically, having the father in the delivery room brings a couple closer, makes birth easier, and helps the woman avoid unnecessary interventions because the father can act as her advocate.

Dr. Michel Odent, a French obstetrician who has delivered over fifteen thousand babies, has a different opinion. He feels that the man's presence actually makes the woman nervous, resulting in longer and more painful labors. He observed that for the man, there is a reaction to seeing his partner in pain that can trigger a chain of events that eventually leads to problems with sexual intimacy in the future.[6]

While there are no definitive studies on this topic, many OBs agree that the father's presence isn't always helpful. Women in labor need to be in a private space where they don't have to think or talk. Having the dad present can change that. Often a woman cannot relax because her partner is anxious. One theory about the rising cesarean rates since the 1970s is that women aren't comfortable with their partner in the room and their labor stalls.

Has society gone too far in expecting all fathers to be present at the birth?

Of course, every couple is different. What may be the societal norm doesn't work for everyone. Your partner may not be the baby's biological father or simply may feel uncomfortable about being present during the delivery. You should discuss whether or how your partner will be involved in your baby's birth before you are in labor. Ideally, your partner's presence strengthens your bond and is a wonderful, lasting memory.

the doctor's diary

I've seen many dads who are happy to meet their baby right after the birth but aren't exactly thrilled to be present throughout the whole process. They often look lost, not knowing how to help and being chastised for even trying. Partners should have a conversation (or two) beforehand to talk about what may be helpful: massage, getting water, or sometimes just staying out of the way. The traditional job of the partner—cutting the cord—isn't always welcomed. I have handed a pair of scissors to a new dad who looks terrified that he is going to hurt the baby. He gives the scissors back to me and asks that I do it myself.

I find female partners behave similarly to fathers, unless they've had a baby themselves. Then, they have the inside track!

The Art of Pushing

Unfortunately, most babies, especially first babies, won't come out on their own for many hours. A significant amount of maternal effort is required to push the baby through the birth canal. And unlike in the movies, the work is much harder than just a few pushes and screams.

The average duration of the second stage of labor for a first time mom without an epidural is thirty-six minutes; twelve minutes for a woman who has had a baby before. With an epidural, it increases to ninety minutes. However, for some unfortunate moms, the second stage can last up to four hours!

Immediate Versus Delayed Pushing

Traditionally, once the cervix has dilated to 10 cm, you would be instructed by your nurse or doctor to start pushing. However, pushing as soon as the cervix is completely open often means that you have a long way to go since the baby may still be high in the pelvis. Delayed pushing, also called laboring down, is waiting to push until your uterus moves the baby lower in the birth canal and your urge to push is stronger. Delayed pushing increases the length of the second stage by almost an hour but decreases the total amount of time you are pushing. Your chance of having a successful vaginal delivery is higher. Especially if you have an epidural, you may not feel the urge to push until the head is quite low and you can allow the force of the uterine contractions to do most of the work.

Mechanics of Pushing

The reason that a baby doesn't fall out of the vagina is the tension in the pelvic floor muscles and vaginal walls. Women who have very rapid labors don't have stronger contractions but have more stretchable pelvic floor muscles.

You will feel a unique urge to push—similar to the feeling that you need to have a bowel movement—as the pressure of the baby's head stimulates the sacral and obturator nerves, which run through the lower part of the pelvis and vagina. The cervix can be fully dilated but you may not yet feel this urge because the head is not low enough to apply pressure on these nerves. Other times, if the baby has descended significantly or is occiput posterior, you may feel the need to push although the cervix isn't fully dilated. Most providers will instruct you not to push until you have reached 10 cm in fear of tearing the cervix, but there is little evidence that this is a significant risk.

Contractions alone have enough force to deliver a baby eventually. However, without maternal effort, it takes a very long time.

When a woman pushes, she contracts her abdominal muscles (rectus), diaphragm, and the muscles between her ribs. This increases the pressure within her abdominal cavity and nearly doubles the downward force to move the baby.

For some women, making grunting or groaning sounds may be helpful as they push. Other women feel better holding their breath.

Pushing Patterns

Directing a woman when to push, when not to push, and how to push has become the norm during childbirth, especially in the hospital setting. Midwives tend to allow women to push instinctively instead of coaching them.

Coached pushing: A common pushing pattern used in the hospital setting is the triple push. In this model, the first push begins as a contraction starts, the second push is at the peak, and third push is while the contraction fades. The nurse will ask the mother to take a breath, hold it, and push while she counts to ten. Then the mother will release the force, push for another ten seconds, and then repeat a third time.

Instinctive pushing: When a woman is allowed to push using her own instincts, she feels the strongest urge near the peak of the contraction, so the push occurs at this point. The baby moves the farthest when the push occurs at the contraction peak. The force of this push is 25 percent greater than pushing outside the peak of the contraction.

Delivery using the triple-push pattern occurs faster (about a nine-minute difference) than when a woman pushes instinctively. However, the total number of pushes is significantly higher (61 percent more pushes) for women doing the triple push.[7] Mothers will need more effort and energy to deliver with the triple push. For women who are tired, pushing instinctively will be easier.

Pushing Positions

The earliest records of childbirth are illustrated with pictures of women delivering in a variety of birthing positions: kneeling, sitting, standing, or squatting. The Babylonian birthing chair from 2000 BC allowed women to sit completely upright. In 1668, Dr. François Mauriceau, a French obstetrician, claimed that reclining on the back with the head and shoulders slightly raised would be easier and more comfortable for the woman and her doctor. Around the world, only 18 percent use a lying-down position for birth, while in the United States, 92 percent of women deliver this way.

The easiest delivery occurs when the hips are slightly flexed, since the pubic bone rotates and the sacrum flattens out. The pelvic outlet, the narrowest part of the pelvis, actually widens about 5 mm in this position. While this may seem like a small amount, every millimeter makes a big difference for a baby navigating the birth canal. Hip flexion can be accomplished in many positions, such as squatting, balancing on hands and knees, or sitting.

For a woman with an epidural, alternative positions are more difficult. While she may be able to move her legs, they usually don't have enough strength to support her weight in a hands and knees or squatting position.

Dorsal lithotomy: Dorsal lithotomy is when a woman lies on her back with her legs separated and feet in stirrups. The doctor has the best access to the baby, so he can guide its delivery. In addition, he can support the perineum with one hand to prevent tears. However, in this position, the sacrum moves forward and reduces the space of the pelvic outlet.

Hands and knees: A woman balances on her hands and knees on a comfortable surface. Gravity pulls the baby toward the floor and creates more space near the sacrum. This position may be most helpful for a baby in the occiput posterior position that needs to rotate.

Lying on her side: While lying on her side, a woman doesn't have to support her weight and can fully relax during a long labor. This position minimizes muscular effort so she can rest between contractions.

Upright: Sitting, squatting, and standing take advantage of the force of gravity and lead to a shorter and less painful second stage of labor than does dorsal lithotomy. These positions move the uterus forward so it is best lined up with the pelvic outlet. In particular, squatting enlarges the pelvis 25 percent more than any other position. However, it can be difficult to balance in a squat on flat feet, so it is important to have something that you can use to prop yourself up, such as a pillow or bolster. Some facilities also offer a squat bar that attaches to a bed. Squatting decreases the duration of the second stage by twenty-three minutes, and is associated with fewer episiotomies and lacerations.[8]

Positions for Crowning

Pulling the legs back during crowning (when the baby's head starts to come out) is a common maneuver used for women who are delivering in dorsal lithotomy. However, this maneuver tightens the skin of the perineum and leads to more lacerations. Letting the legs down in normal, relaxed position decreases this tension.

the doctor's diary

Trust me when I say that a doctor's goal is to have the baby come out easily, safely, and quickly. The last thing I want is to spend hours pushing with a patient who is not making any progress. You would think doctors would do whatever it takes to get the baby out faster. If a certain position would make it easier, it would be logical that doctors would suggest it.

However, in residency, I was trained to deliver babies with the woman on her back and feet in stirrups—the dorsal lithotomy position. I delivered hundreds of babies like this. I was taught that the pelvis is a fixed, bony structure whose size does not change with position. I believed the dorsal lithotomy was best, because it allows the head and shoulders to squeeze under the pubic bone easily and allows room to work in case a baby gets stuck. However, recent studies show that the pelvic size, with its flexible ligaments, widens in certain positions, such as squatting and sitting, and these positions may actually provide a few extra millimeters of opening for the baby to get through.

I remember the first time I had a patient who wanted to deliver in a position other than dorsal lithotomy. I was two years into my private practice and had delivered over one thousand patients on their back. She came into the hospital in active labor, desiring a natural delivery. Her back pain prevented her from lying down comfortably, so she got on all fours in the bed. She began to push in this position, on her hands and knees. Honestly, I couldn't get oriented. I was accustomed to helping to stretch the perineum in a downward direction, but now down was up. I would normally guide the baby's head out by applying slight downward traction to release the shoulder from under the pubic bone, but now the pubic bone was on top. But as it turned out, the baby and mom were able to figure things out without my help. The baby's head naturally stretched the perineum and the mother's effort pushed the baby right under the bone with no problem.

Most doctors still insist on their patients using the dorsal lithotomy position. Some natural birthing advocates say this birthing position is for the doctor's convenience. I wouldn't call it convenience per se—it is actually because the other positions are simply unfamiliar. Laboring mothers need to insist on positions that feel comfortable for them. Residents in training should learn about these alternate birthing positions from the beginning, so they can support what works best for their patient.

Clamping and Cutting the Cord

Once the baby has delivered, the next step is cutting the umbilical cord. Traditionally, the cord is clamped and cut within a minute of birth. Immediately cutting the cord allows the third stage of labor to progress faster, decreases the risk of maternal hemorrhage, and decreases the risk of jaundice in the newborn. However, delaying cord clamping for three to five minutes allows an additional 3 to 4 ounces of blood to move from the placenta to the baby, improving iron stores in the newborn and decreasing the risk of anemia. This "placental transfusion" is especially important for preemies and for infants who will be breastfed because iron levels in breast milk are low. Delayed cord clamping also helps to maintain newborn blood pressure and assists with the transition to air breathing.

Ideally, the baby should be positioned near the level of the placenta for at least three minutes before clamping and cutting the cord. Lifting the baby more than 7 inches above the placenta significantly reduces or reverses the flow of blood. The perfect position for the baby is on its mother's chest.

The cord may need to be cut immediately if it is tightly wrapped around the baby's neck and prevents the baby from coming out. If a baby is under significant distress at the time of delivery and needs immediate attention and resuscitation, the cord will also need to be cut right away. Collecting cord blood for banking may preclude waiting to cut the cord as well. If most of the blood flows into the baby, there won't be enough for adequate cord blood storage.

CORD BLOOD BANKING: THE TRUTH ABOUT CORD BLOOD TRANSPLANTS

Cord blood is the blood that remains in the umbilical cord and placenta after the baby has delivered. This blood contains stem cells that can grow into mature blood cells. Stem cells are unique in that they have fewer proteins on their surface so they are easier to match to a transplant recipient. Cord blood banking is done to store these stem cells for use as a treatment for certain diseases that the baby or another family member may develop later in life. In 2014, 1.4 million parents banked their baby's cord blood, making this a $3 billion per year industry.

Umbilical cord stem cells should not be confused with embryonic stem cells. Cord blood cells only grow into red and white blood cells

continues–

—continued

that can be used to treat leukemia and anemia. Embryonic cells develop into any cell type in the body and can be used for regenerative medicine, such as the treatment of spinal cord injuries or Parkinson's disease. Bone marrow is the other source of immature blood cells that is traditionally used to treat leukemias and anemias. However, it must be obtained through a surgical procedure and transplants require a perfect match between donor and recipient.

Cord blood is easy to collect and poses no risk to the mother or baby. You may need to forgo delayed cord clamping so as to get enough blood. The chance of using your banked blood is 1 in 100,000. There were 4,626 transplants between 2008 and 2013 in the United States. Of these, 9 percent were given to the donor, 2 percent to a relative, and 89 percent to a person unrelated to the donor.[9]

Most cord blood samples (75 percent) are too small to be used by anyone because they don't contain enough stem cells. Cord blood can only be used if the recipient weighs less than 90 pounds, limiting its use to children.

More than twenty private cord blood banks exist in the United States. They advertise everywhere, in pregnancy magazines, online, and in doctors' offices. They suggest that cord blood stem cells may have the potential to cure such diseases as autism, Alzheimer's, or diabetes someday, but these claims are purely hypothetical. Cord blood companies charge about $2,000 with an annual storage fee of $200.

The American College of Obstetricians and Gynecologists and the American Academy of Pediatrics discourage patients from using private banks, unless they already have a sick child who might benefit from the blood. Instead, women are encouraged to use public banks so that treatments with cord blood are available to all patients, regardless of their ability to pay for it.

Be the Match Registry lists bone marrow donors and donated umbilical cord blood units. Donating your baby's cord blood to a public bank is free. On the website www.bethematch.org, you can find out whether your hospital is affiliated with a public cord blood bank.

the doctor's diary

Twenty-nine states have laws that either encourage or require providers to discuss cord blood options with their patients. We must inform patients that the blood can be banked privately, publicly, or discarded.

Many representatives of cord blood banks don't make it clear to patients that, if their child has a disorder, the blood probably can't be used for that child or any other recipient because the stem cells would also be affected. In addition, cord blood is not the first line of treatment for most diseases. Instead, oncologists will choose a known approach, such as chemotherapy, that has a proven track record.

Cord blood companies directly pressure patients to commit to banking cord blood. A patient told me that she called a company for more information but decided against it. She received seven phone calls from the company over the next few months, suggesting that she "do this out of love and responsibility for your family." Of course, a mom would do anything she can to protect her baby. Cord blood storage companies capitalize on this sentiment. Instead of falling for the sales pressure, I would recommend to find a public bank where your cord blood can be used for anyone in need.

The Third Stage of Labor

The average duration of the third stage of labor, from delivery of the baby to delivery of the placenta, is six minutes. Oxytocin continues to stimulate uterine contractions that cause the placenta to separate from the wall of the uterus. The large blood vessels that delivered nutrients and oxygen to the fetus quickly constrict, limiting blood loss. In three percent of births, the placenta doesn't detach properly or the blood vessels fail to constrict, and a postpartum hemorrhage (PPH) occurs. PPH is the most common cause of maternal death worldwide. Women who are at highest risk of PPH are those with a long labor, large baby, or twins, or those who have given birth many times before.

Options for the Third Stage

In nearly all hospital births, after the baby has delivered, Pitocin is immediately given and the cord is cut. Traction is applied to the cord to hasten delivery of the placenta and, once it is out, the uterus is massaged. Many new moms aren't even aware that these events are taking place because they happen within minutes. These actions reduce the risk of PPH by 68 percent but have side effects, such as nausea, headaches, and pain from the uterine massage.

If you are unlikely to bleed excessively, your provider may agree to forgo these traditional interventions. Instead, she can delay clamping the cord, avoid using Pitocin, and deliver the placenta with the assistance of gravity instead of cord traction. Stimulating the release of natural oxytocin by the newborn sucking at the breast and by being in an environment with low lighting, warmth, and comfort can help to control postpartum bleeding. Of course, if your bleeding is more than normal, medications can be given to decrease it, whether you delivered in a hospital, birthing center, or at home.

Lotus Birth

Lotus birth is the term for a birth in which the umbilical cord is never cut. Instead, the cord and placenta are left to fall off naturally in three to ten days. Usually, the placenta is wrapped in a towel and laid next to the baby.

---

the doctor's diary

Medically, I can't find a reason that a Lotus birth is superior to delayed cord clamping. All the placental blood transfers to the baby within the first few minutes after delivery, at which time the remaining blood in the cord naturally clots. No additional nutrients are passed to the newborn after this point. One nonmedical advantage may be that a baby is less likely to be disturbed by being passed around to family and friends if it has a placenta still attached, encouraging time alone for mother and baby.

The detached placenta is a mixture of tissue and blood that may be the perfect breeding ground for bacteria. However, because the number of Lotus births is low, there are no studies on the incidence of infection.

When you have your first contraction, we know what the final outcome is likely to be. One way or another, you will have a baby in your arms. But the hours or days that you will be in labor are packed with new experiences and surprises. While the mechanics of labor are similar for all women—one stage following another—your experience will be uniquely your own.

INTERVENTIONS IN THE DELIVERY ROOM: EXCEPTION OR RULE?

MEDICAL INTERVENTIONS DURING LABOR HAVE SAVED MILLIONS of lives. Better hygiene prevents infection, medications stop bleeding, cesareans rescue babies from mothers in a medical crisis. Emergencies arise, and the full extent of scientific breakthroughs keeps mothers and babies safe.

the doctor's diary

While in medical school, I volunteered at St. Jude Hospital on the Caribbean island of Saint Lucia. St. Jude's had almost no modern equipment but provided basic care to the island residents who paid for medical services with fruit, goats, and chickens. I felt as if I had been transported into the past.

We had one fetal monitor in the maternity area that would be shared among all the women. I remember one woman who was enduring a particularly long labor. I placed the monitor on her abdomen and found that her baby's heartbeat was dangerously low. She needed a cesarean and she needed it quickly. But there was no anesthesiologist. I had no choices that a modern hospital offers. Sadly, her baby was lost. Without a doubt, this child would have survived with medical intervention.

Lifesaving procedures in obstetrics that were meant to be the exceptions have now become the rule. Laboring women with low-risk pregnancies are treated the same as those who are high risk. One intervention often leads to many more. Although 60 percent of women say they prefer to have no medical interventions, only 17 percent achieve this goal.[1] In the United States:

- 80% have an IV.
- 70% use an epidural.
- 60% are not allowed to move around or walk during labor.
- 65% have a urinary catheter.
- 31% receive Pitocin.
- 32% deliver by a cesarean.
- 30% are induced.
- 65% have their water broken artificially.
- 94% have continuous fetal monitoring.

Cesarean

A cesarean section (commonly known as a C-section) is a surgical birth performed when a medical situation exists that, if labor were to continue, would put the mother's or baby's life at risk. The cesarean is the most common operation in the United States. One third of the deliveries in the nation, over 1.3 million every year, are cesareans. There is no doubt that cesareans save lives in a true emergency. But numerous cesareans are done because one was done with a previous birth, because of the fear of ending up with one anyway after a prolonged labor, or because of impatience on the part of the family or the doctor—or both.

The use of cesareans has increased by 500 percent since 1970. Twenty percent are scheduled in advance because a woman has had one previously, and 80 percent happen in first-time births. The C-section rate varies widely from state to state, from a low of 22 percent in Utah to 39 percent in Louisiana, suggesting that there are regional practice patterns that influence the frequency with which cesareans are performed. Cesarean rates are influenced by other factors, such as convenience, perceived safety, medical training of physicians, and fear of litigation.

Some have hypothesized that the higher rates today are due to an increase in the number of older women with more complicated pregnancies, but the rates are actually higher for women of all ages. In fact, for healthy women under the age of twenty-five, the C-section rate has increased by 57 percent in the last two decades.

High cesarean rates have become an international phenomenon. In Brazil, over 85 percent of births in private hospitals are by C-section; here, the fear of the pain of childbirth is passed down from generation to generation and women are warned that their body will be permanently damaged by a vaginal delivery. Many Brazilian physicians also suggest cesareans for vague reasons that mostly have to do with their own convenience. The lowest cesarean rates in the world are in Africa, where only 5 percent of babies are born surgically. An analysis of childbirth in 194 countries suggests that the "ideal" rate of cesareans should be 19 percent. When the rate is in this range, maternal and newborn deaths decline. When the rate exceeds this, there is no increased benefit to the mother or baby and instead there may be complications from unnecessary surgeries.[2] Of course, cesareans should be provided to women who need them, and not to achieve any specific rate.

Medical advancements and new technologies have contributed to the increase in the cesarean rate. Continuous electronic fetal monitoring during labor may show changes in a baby's heart rate that suggest it may be stressed, prompting a cesarean to be performed. However, in most cases, the baby is perfectly fine. Similarly, ultrasounds diagnose "big babies," which lead doctors to recommend cesareans to women without even attempting a vaginal birth.

Doctors find themselves erring on the side of caution and relying on technologies that can't give perfect answers.

> For years, I never knew my exact cesarean rate. I believed that I recommended it when it was justified and necessary. I remember even feeling offended when a patient asked about the rate, as if she was questioning my judgment. However, my attitude changed after researching for this book. I realized it is important for each doctor to know their rate and how it compares to that of other doctors with similar practices. It turns out that my rate was slightly lower than average.

Most hospitals keep track of their individual doctors' cesarean rates, but the data collected are for their use only. The Joint Commission on Accreditation of Healthcare Organizations (JCAHO) requires that all hospitals with more than 1,100 births per year calculate their cesarean section rates. In this way, a hospital can see where it stands among similar institutions. However, this information is also not made public. About half of US hospitals voluntarily report their data to organizations that advocate for patient safety. The cesarean rates for specific hospitals, but not individual doctors, can be found at the Leapfrog Group: www.leapfroggroup.org /compare-hospitals.

Hospitals do not create protocols to keep cesarean rates at a certain level. If a doctor has a higher-than-average rate, the administration assumes it is because that doctor takes care of more high-risk patients. When a doctor decides to perform a cesarean, there isn't another doctor or hospital administrator validating his decision.

Hospitals that employ laborists have cesarean rates 25 to 30 percent lower than do those with the traditional private practice model. This suggests that one quarter of cesareans are likely done for the convenience of the doctor, who often cites the reason for surgery as a "failure to progress," when it is more likely a "failure to wait" on the part of the doctor.

the doctor's diary

While the laborist model decreases the cesarean rate, it also changes the dynamics of prenatal care. As an obstetrician, one of my greatest joys is sharing the experience of childbirth with a woman I know well. I know her fears and desires about the birth and relish the unique relationship we've established. I didn't choose this field for the lifestyle; I chose it because I enjoy getting to know a patient throughout many stages of life, including pregnancy.

As an OB, I want to believe that my patients prefer for me to be at their delivery. But surveys of patients delivered by laborists show something different. Most women are looking for a positive birth experience with whoever is there. They want to be heard, to be part of the decision-making process, and to have the delivery they want—whether that is a natural birth, a birth with medication, or a cesarean. High levels of satisfaction with the laborist model shows us that the person attending the delivery doesn't have to be known; he just has to be open and supportive.

Who Has Cesareans

Women who are more likely to deliver by cesarean are:

- Older
- Caucasian
- Having their first baby
- Wealthier
- Diabetic
- Hypertensive
- Obese

the doctor's diary

Failure to perform a cesarean is one of the most common reasons that an OB is sued for malpractice. Doctors want to deliver the baby before there is a bad outcome. But our ability to predict bad outcomes is limited. Once a cesarean is done, we will never know what would have happened if we had waited. Most doctors believe it is better to err on the side of caution and feel that they can defend themselves in a lawsuit by showing they took action to protect the baby. Early in residency, we are taught that you can never be blamed for doing a cesarean, only blamed for not doing one.

Reasons for Cesareans

- Dystocia (the baby isn't coming out). This can be due to arrest of dilation or arrest of descent.
- Fetal distress
- Breech
- Twins
- Large baby

Situations Where a Cesarean Is the Only Option

The following situations mandate a cesarean delivery. If these occur when a woman is under the care of a midwife, she will be immediately transferred to a doctor.

- Placenta previa
- Uterine rupture
- Cord prolapse
- Active herpes outbreak
- Transverse fetus (lying sideways)

Benefits of a Cesarean for the Baby

- Safe and prompt delivery of the baby
- Eliminates the risk of shoulder dystocia and associated birth injuries

- Eliminates the chance of brain damage due to severe fetal distress during labor

Risks of a Cesarean for the Baby

While a cesarean may be the safest way to give birth to a healthy baby in certain circumstances, it is not without its own risks. During pregnancy, the fetal lungs are filled with amniotic fluid. This fluid must be cleared after delivery so that the baby can breathe air. In a vaginal birth, some of this fluid is squeezed out of the baby's mouth and nose as it passes through the birth canal. In a cesarean, this doesn't happen, and the baby may have difficulty breathing, a condition called transient tachypnea of the newborn (TTN). Although TTN is usually not a long-term problem, the baby may need to be separated from its family in the NICU for a number of days.

Traveling through the birth canal also exposes a baby to bacteria from its mother's genital tract. These bacteria that colonize the newborn's intestines are responsible for digestion, immunity, and disease prevention. Babies born by cesarean, especially those whose mothers did not labor, become colonized with different bacteria. Doctors believe this may be why cesarean babies have an increased risk of digestive issues, ear and respiratory infections, allergies, obesity, and diabetes.

Seeding a C-section baby with these good bacteria is a new trend. Swabbing a newborn with bacteria from its mother's genital tract can introduce the bacteria they would have received if born vaginally, possibly lowering the risk of illnesses.[3] As long as the mother does not have any infections, such as HIV, chlamydia, herpes, or Group B strep, there does not appear to be any risk. To seed your baby, insert a sterile gauze in your vagina for one hour before your cesarean. After birth, wipe your newborn's mouth, face, and hands with the gauze. The procedure is only suggested for women who were not in labor, such as those who have a cesarean scheduled because of a breech baby or preeclampsia.

Benefits of Cesarean for the Mother

- Avoidance of the pain and unknowns of labor
- Decreased risk of urinary incontinence
- Convenience
- Elimination of vaginal trauma

Risk of Cesarean for the Mother

- Blood clots: The risk of developing a blood clot is 4 times higher with a cesarean birth than with a vaginal delivery.
- Maternal death: 3.6 per 100,000 with vaginal birth; 5.9 per 100,000 with scheduled cesarean, 18.2 per 100,000 with emergency cesarean.
- Injury to organs near the uterus: Bowel or bladder
- Bleeding: The average blood loss with a vaginal delivery is 300 cc; with a cesarean, 600 cc.
- Longer and more painful recovery
- Wound infections
- Higher cost
- Development of scar tissue in the abdomen, which can lead to bowel obstruction

Scheduling a Cesarean

Most cesareans are a result of something that happens during labor. However, some are scheduled ahead of time. A planned cesarean should be done only after you have reached thirty-nine weeks, to ensure that your baby is fully mature. Cesareans are often scheduled for breech babies, twins, and placenta previas and for women who have had a cesarean before.

If you know that you will be delivering by cesarean, most doctors will insist on picking your surgery date (usually at thirty-nine weeks) a month or two ahead of time. However, allowing spontaneous labor to begin and then proceeding with surgery may be beneficial to your baby. Even a few hours of contractions decrease the chance of breathing problems in the newborn and improves breastfeeding success.[4] In addition, if your water breaks, natural seeding with the good bacteria takes place.

So, why do doctors prefer to schedule cesareans? I hate to admit it, but it is all about convenience. Your labor may kick in during the middle of the night, when the doctor is in another surgery, or when he is in the office with other patients. These scheduled cesareans make a doctor's life more manageable.

If you prefer to wait for spontaneous labor before having your surgery, ask your doctor whether this is an option. If you are delivering at a hospital that utilizes laborists, it may be very easy to fulfil this request. If you have a placenta previa or your baby is in footling breech presentation, you should not wait for labor to begin, as these situations can have dangerous complications.

How Future Pregnancies Are Affected by a Previous Cesarean

Having a cesarean greatly impacts your future pregnancies. Your chance of ever having a vaginal birth decreases because many doctors and hospitals no longer allow VBAC (vaginal birth after cesarean). Placenta accreta, when the placenta grows into the uterine scar, and uterine rupture, in which the uterine scar opens during labor, are complications specific to women who have had cesareans in the past. In addition, as with all surgeries, scar tissue can develop after a cesarean leading to bowel obstruction and pain. This scar tissue also makes future cesareans technically difficult.

If Your Doctor Recommends a Cesarean

- Make sure you have a clear understanding of the reason.

- Ask whether there are any alternatives.
- Ask whether this is an emergency.
- Don't panic. While it may not be the birth you dreamed of, it can still be a beautiful experience. You should focus on the fact that it will only be a few minutes before you meet your baby. Now, in some facilities, you can have skin-to-skin contact with your baby in the OR.

Legally, you can refuse a cesarean. You cannot be compelled to have any medical procedure for the benefit of another person—in this case, your baby. The American College of Obstetricians and Gynecologists (ACOG) agrees that seeking a court order to force a woman to have a cesarean is unethical. It is the duty of your doctor to explain fully why a cesarean is necessary and to bring in other physicians for second and third opinions. But he can never perform a cesarean without your consent unless it is a true emergency in which you are unable to give consent or are not capable of understanding what is going on, such as in the case of a patient who has lost consciousness. Despite this legal framework, there have been cases where women have been forced to have surgery, who have been picked up from home by police, or had their babies taken away by social workers. Thankfully, these situations are very rare.

the doctor's diary

Many patients tell me at their first prenatal visit that, no matter what, they don't want a cesarean. However, it's not really something you can opt out of in advance. In most cases, the decision to have a cesarean is not made until you are in labor. But there are things you can do during pregnancy to keep yourself fit and healthy so that a cesarean becomes less likely. You should exercise regularly and avoid gaining an excessive amount of weight. Allow labor to start on its own. Arrive at the hospital only once you are in active labor. If you are admitted to the hospital before you have reached 4 cm, you have an increased risk of epidural and Pitocin use as well as a higher chance of a cesarean.

❧ CHRISTINE'S STORY ❧

Christine was pleasantly surprised about her experience having an unplanned cesarean. She was a healthy, twenty-nine-year-old TV writer who had planned on a noninterventional birth. She had taken the twelve-week Bradley birthing course and hired a doula. Christine went into labor at thirty-eight weeks. Her doula came to her home for the first few hours to help her through the early phase. When they arrived at the hospital, she was 4 cm dilated. Her baby's heart rate looked great, so she was allowed to walk around the room. She was breathing and moaning through the contractions with the help of her doula and husband. Her water broke on its own, and the pain became much more intense; nearly unbearable. However, the baby's heart rate suddenly became very low. With every contraction, her baby's heartbeat dropped. I examined her and could feel that a small loop of the umbilical cord was next to the baby's head. When she had a contraction, the uterus was squeezing on this loop and the heart rate would drop. I tried to push the cord out of the way, but to no avail. Christine needed a cesarean quickly.

After I explained what was happening, we hurriedly prepared her for surgery. Christine looked so disappointed—everything had been going perfectly. Once in the OR, her husband and doula joined her. We put on the music that she was playing in her labor room. The anesthesiologist placed her spinal, and immediately the pain from the contractions was gone.

Then something changed in her mind-set. Christine decided to look at this experience as something new and interesting. She was asking all sorts of questions, such as how the anesthesia works and what the different monitors in the OR are for. She was truly fascinated by what was going on. She asked me to tell her what I was seeing as I did her surgery. She viewed it as a unique opportunity to be wide awake during a surgical procedure and to appreciate the advances of modern medicine. I commented on her strong abdominal muscles, her beautiful ovaries, and, of course, the details of her baby's face. It was like giving a play-by-play. I told her about the type of suture we used to close the opening in the uterus, how we sew up the skin, and what she would feel like over the next few days. Christine took the turn of events in stride and made it educational for herself. Afterward, she said she had no regrets—she was able to experience labor. She felt confident that she had done nothing wrong that led to her having a cesarean. She was grateful for the opportunity for her baby to be born healthy. ❧

The Elective Cesarean

An elective cesarean is one that is done prior to labor at the request of the mother, when there are no maternal or fetal health concerns. In the United States, about 2 percent of cesareans are elective, accounting for 0.6 percent of all births. A 2001 survey of ob-gyns showed that 32 percent of female OBs would choose an elective cesarean for themselves and 56 percent of the male OBs would choose it for their partners. In some parts of the world, over 15 percent of deliveries are cesareans on request.[5]

ACOG supports a woman's choice to have a cesarean without any medical necessity. Women request cesareans for a variety of reasons: convenience, fear of labor/pain, a previous bad experience in labor, concerns about future urinary incontinence or painful sex.

Whether an elective cesarean is better for a woman and her baby compared to a planned vaginal birth is unclear. There are risks and benefits to both. Of course, most women who decide to have a cesarean will have a healthy baby and recover without complications.

the doctor's diary

If a patient asks me for an elective cesarean, I first try to find out why she wants it. The most common reason is fear of pain, followed by fear of tearing the vagina, fear of incontinence, and simply believing it's not possible. Sometimes, a clear explanation of available pain medications will change her mind. Ultimately, I believe that every woman has the right to choose her birthing style. If she knows and understands the risks and makes an informed decision, whether it is to have a baby at home or to have an elective, scheduled cesarean, I will support her.

Many of my patients say that their fears about childbirth stem from things other doctors have said to them well before they were even pregnant. They describe comments suggesting that they will have trouble delivering a baby. They have been told things like "your pelvis is so small," "your uterus is tipped," "you are so tiny," and so on. These off-the-cuff, inadvertent remarks stick in the back of a woman's mind for years, creating a narrative that becomes a self-fulfilling prophecy. During pregnancy, a doctor may say, "Your baby is big" or "The baby is never going to fit." I don't think doctors understand how much these offhand comments influence their patients' outlook on childbirth. I believe there needs to be a better conversation about a woman's natural ability to give birth. Women need to know that babies are usually made to fit their mothers, that our body is well designed to give birth, and that changes happen to the body during labor that allow the process to be successful.

Experience of a Cesarean

Some women feel pain, nausea, difficulty breathing, and anxiety during the surgery. They may also be surprised (or disappointed) to hear their doctors talking about their weekend plans or how their kids are doing in school while they are prepping for the surgery and during the operation.

There is a higher risk of postpartum depression among women who have had an unplanned cesarean. Women describe a sense of failure and loss of control. Whereas some women see a cesarean as a necessary route to having a healthy baby, others are traumatized by the experience, and feel guilt, shame, embarrassment, or even post-traumatic stress disorder (PTSD). In a recent survey, 25 percent of women say they felt pressured to have a cesarean and 47 percent described it as traumatic. However, many women have had great experiences of a cesarean, especially if it is planned. They go into the hospital, have an IV placed, get a spinal, and thirty minutes later, it's over and they have their baby.

Recovery after a cesarean varies. Some women are up and moving the next day with minimal pain. Others require pain medication, and have difficulty tending to the needs of their baby. Breastfeeding can be more challenging because the baby can't lie comfortably against the mother's incision. Women with scheduled cesareans generally have the easiest time afterward, whereas women who has been in labor for days, pushed for hours, and then had surgery have the slowest recovery.

Labor Induction

When labor doesn't start on its own, medications and other techniques can be used to stimulate contractions. In the United States, 25 to 30 percent of all births are induced, up from 9 percent in 1990. Many inductions are necessary, but 40 percent are elective, meaning there is no medical indication for artificially starting labor.

The hormone progesterone suppresses uterine activity for most of pregnancy. As delivery nears, progesterone levels decline and contractions begin. Waves of muscular contractions pass from the top to the bottom of the uterus, producing large amounts of highly organized energy. This complicated process is extremely difficult to replicate using artificial means. For this reason, induced labor is never exactly the same as spontaneous labor.

An induction bypasses the body's natural preparation for labor that begins weeks earlier, during which time the baby's head rotates into the correct position and the cervix softens. When the baby is not positioned correctly, it will have difficulty progressing through its cardinal movements. Softening of the cervix is accomplished with medications over a few hours instead with natural hormones over a few weeks. In spontaneous labor, endorphins—our natural painkillers—rise throughout labor. In induced labor, endorphin levels remain constant, leading to the increased use of epidurals.

Reasons for Induction

Inductions are done when the doctor determines that it is safer for the baby to be born or it is safer for the mother to no longer be pregnant. The two reasons for induction that have been scientifically proven beneficial for mothers or babies are:

- Postterm pregnancy (after 42 weeks)
- Preeclampsia

Other common reasons for induction that have *not* been proven to be beneficial:

- The mother is uncomfortable.
- The baby is at or near the due date.
- The baby appears large.
- The water has broken but labor hasn't started.
- Maternal convenience with work/childcare
- Low amniotic fluid
- Poor fetal growth (IUGR)
- The mother wants to deliver with a specific provider.

Elective Inductions

An induction without a clear medical reason is called an elective, or "social," induction. It is scheduled at the convenience of doctor, patient, and hospital staff. It allows mothers to arrange childcare for older siblings, plan for time off work, or alleviate the discomfort of late pregnancy. Elective inductions eliminate the fear of not making it to the hospital on time. Elective induction should not be done until at least thirty-nine weeks.

Medical Methods for Inducing Labor

Labor can be induced by using synthetic hormones or mechanical methods. The decision of which method to use depends on the condition of your cervix and the preference of your doctor. Almost all inductions take place in a hospital, but some doctors using the balloon dilator method may start it at home. Inductions must be done under the supervision of a physician, not a midwife.

Pitocin, the synthetic form of oxytocin, is the most common induction agent. It is used when the cervix has already softened and effaced, with a Bishop score of 6 or more (for more about Bishop scores, see page 134). Unlike natural oxytocin from the brain, which is released in a pulse, Pitocin is given as a continuous infusion through an IV that starts at a low dosage level and is increased over time. Pitocin's side effects include headaches, nausea, and painful contractions.

Prostaglandins, such as misoprostol and dinoprostone, are used when the cervix is still firm and thick with a Bishop score of 5 or less. They are administered as a pill, vaginal suppository, or gel. The side effects are nausea, diarrhea, and fevers.

Balloon dilators are used to mechanically open the cervix, causing the release of natural prostaglandins. A rubber balloon is placed into the cervix and inflated. The dilator does not have any side effects but requires that the cervix be slightly open.

Amniotomy, breaking the water bag, causes the release of prostaglandins and can only be done if the cervix is partially open. An amnihook, a plastic stick with a small metal hook on the end that resembles a crochet hook, is threaded through the cervical opening. A sweeping motion moves the hook upward, where the metal end snags the amniotic membrane and breaks it. Once the water bag is broken, vaginal bacteria can travel into the uterus, causing infections in the mother or newborn.

Risks of Induced Labor

Labor induction can lead to a cascade of other medical interventions. You must stay in bed with an IV and continuous fetal monitoring. The contractions feel more painful since you can't move around and endorphins aren't released naturally. As a result, you are more likely to want or need an epidural. Pushing can be more challenging with an epidural, and therefore, you may need a cesarean.

	Epidural rate	Cesarean rate
Induced labor	78%	28%
Spontaneous labor	61%	13%[6]

Excessive uterine contractions can occur with the medications Pitocin and prostaglandins. In 5 to 10 percent of inductions, having contractions that are too strong or too frequent diminishes the oxygen flow to the baby, a phenomenon called hyperstimulation. This may lead to fetal distress and a cesarean. In addition, induced labors last longer and the total time spent in the hospital is greater, increasing health care costs.

the doctor's diary

Without a doubt, elective inductions are convenient for doctors. If a patient mentioned that she was tired, uncomfortable, and just couldn't stand being pregnant anymore, I would happily schedule a delivery date for her. One of the first things you learn as a new doctor in private practice is when to start an induction so your patient delivers during daytime hours. The timing is truly an art! You take into consideration how many babies the patient has had, the cervical dilation, effacement, and so on. However, after practicing for years, I realize that these elective inductions are only for convenience and result in longer hospital stays than spontaneous labor. In some cases, they don't work at all, and a woman has an unnecessary cesarean.

Deemphasizing due dates is one way to cut down on elective inductions. I find that some women focus on that day and don't want to be pregnant a minute longer. Thinking of a delivery window as lasting for four to five weeks will help women feel more comfortable staying pregnant until nature takes its course.

Factors That Influence Whether an Induction Will Be Successful

- If you have had a baby before, your chance of having a successful induction is seven times higher than if you've never had a baby.
- If your Bishop score is higher than 7, the success rate is the same as spontaneous labor.
- If your Bishop score is lower than 7, the cesarean rate after induced labor is 32 percent.

Alternatives for Induction

Unfortunately, if an induction is deemed necessary, few nonmedical options will get labor started. You may read articles and websites that tout numerous methods. Even doctors and midwives may suggest more natural procedures, but none has ever proven effective:

- Acupuncture: Results of studies are inconclusive on the use of acupuncture to induce labor.
- Breast stimulation: This causes the release of natural oxytocin. Massaging the breasts or applying warm compresses three times per day is most helpful in women with high Bishop scores.
- Castor oil: Castor oil is a laxative that stimulates the production of natural prostaglandins. However, it also brings on diarrhea and nausea. No formal studies have been conducted on its ability to induce labor, but it definitely will keep you in the bathroom for most of the night.
- Evening primrose oil (EPO): This contains linolenic acid, which stimulates the production of prostaglandins. While evidence of its effectiveness is only anecdotal, it does appear to be safe. Women take two or three 500 mg capsules daily, starting at thirty-six weeks.
- Membrane stripping: To strip the membranes, your provider inserts a finger through the open cervix and moves it in a circular motion to detach the membrane of the water bag from the uterine wall. Weekly membrane stripping in the last few weeks of pregnancy reduces the need for induction and lowers the chance of being postterm, but hasn't been proven as an induction agent itself. While it is not dangerous, even in women who are GBS carriers, it is quite uncomfortable. In some cases, your provider may be stripping your membranes without your even knowing it during a routine cervical exam.

- Red raspberry leaf tea: This tea, used safely since the sixth century, is thought to prepare the uterus for labor. Most studies show it does not induce labor, but may help decrease the length of the second stage by up to ten minutes and make labor easier.
- Sex: Sex causes the local release of prostaglandins. However, most studies do not show it to be effective at inducing labor.
- Spicy foods: Eating spicy foods does not bring on labor.
- Walking: Walking does not make labor start but being upright and moving allows the baby to settle lower into the birth canal.

WARNING

Black cohosh makes contractions more effective. However, it also thins the blood, increasing blood loss at delivery so it is *not recommended*.

Blue cohosh makes contractions stronger but it may also affect heart muscle activity so it is *not recommended*.

Amniotomy (Artificial Rupture of Membranes, or AROM)

Amniotomy, also known as artificial rupture of membranes (AROM), is performed in 65 percent of pregnancies as a means to induce labor (see page 230) or to speed along a spontaneous labor, making it one of the most common medical interventions. In theory, removing the soft cushion of the amniotic sac allows the hard head of the baby to push against the cervix and dilate it more effectively. Like membrane stripping, it also releases natural prostaglandins. However, the duration of labor is essentially the same with and without amniotomy. The only legitimate reason that an amniotomy should be performed in spontaneous labor is if a woman requires internal, continuous fetal monitoring with a scalp electrode or uterine pressure catheter.[7] Internal monitoring is done when external monitoring is technically difficult, such as in the case of an obese woman.

Disadvantages to AROM

- Higher cesarean rate for first-time mothers: Because the cushion around the baby is gone, it is more difficult to rotate into the correct position and proceed through the cardinal movements.
- Cord compression: When the fluid around the baby is low, the umbilical cord can be compressed during contractions, leading to fetal distress.
- Rapid transition to painful labor: Within minutes of AROM, mild contractions can transition into intense pain. Feeling unprepared for this sudden shift, some patients may become discouraged or distraught.
- Fetal infections: Once the water has broken, bacteria can travel into the uterus. Women are now "on the clock" and need to deliver in a certain amount of time to minimize the risk of fetal infections.

the doctor's diary

Amniotomy has been a routine practice in the United States and many other countries around the world for years. As a resident, I was taught that as soon as I could get a finger or two in the cervix, I should break the water to expedite the labor. I assumed that women would want to deliver as quickly as possible. When I saw women's pain and frequency of contractions increase so dramatically after AROM, it seemed to be a good thing—that labor would progress faster. However, my assumption was far from the truth for many of my patients. When they were not prepared for the change in contraction intensity, they would lose control and would change their entire birth plan on the spot. And as many studies have shown, amniotomy does not make the labor go any faster.

When the water drains from the uterus, the umbilical cord can be compressed, which leads to variable decelerations. We treat this fetal heart rate pattern by putting water back into the uterus through a small tube, called an amnioinfusion. I remember one patient asking me, "Why did you just let the water out only to put it back in ten minutes later?" This is an excellent question!

I hope that amniotomy will be one of those interventions, like routine episiotomy and enemas, that will eventually go by the wayside. If your doctor suggests it, ask her why. It is your right to decline if there doesn't seem to be a clear reason.

Use of IVs

Intravenous fluids are given routinely during 80 percent of labors in the United States to prevent dehydration and to correct low blood pressure that can result from an epidural. The fluids run at 125 to 250 cc per hour, which amounts to 3 to 6 liters in a 24-hour period. It's no wonder patients are swollen after delivery!

Labor, like any exercise, requires hydration. Women who are not eating or drinking deliver quicker if they receive IV fluids. However, those who stay hydrated by drinking aren't benefited by the additional IV. Women instinctively know when and how much to drink during labor. Therefore, using an IV in a healthy woman who is able to eat and drink is not necessary.

An IV is uncomfortable and it limits your movements. Women giving birth at home or in a birthing center rarely have an IV. In the hospital setting, your doctor may agree to waive the IV fluids if you have a saline lock. A saline lock is a 2-inch plastic tube that is placed into a vein and taped to your arm. It allows full mobility because IV tubing isn't connected to it. The saline lock can easily be connected to IV tubing and fluids if you want pain medication, such as an epidural or narcotics, or need fluids due to unexpected blood loss. Like a regular IV, the saline lock may feel uncomfortable in the arm and can cause some local bruising.

Eating and Drinking During Labor

Most women, 76 percent, are not allowed to eat or drink while in labor. This rule was based on a 1946 study that showed that laboring women were prone to aspiration (when a woman vomits and breathes it into her lungs).[8] However, women in this study were completely sedated, unlike women today who are awake. Today, the risk of aspiration is 0.6 per million—calling into question the necessity of this rule.

Eating is usually done in the latent phase of labor. In active labor and while pushing, food is the last thing on your mind. However, drinking should continue to avoid dehydration. The natural approach—and that taken by most midwives especially at home and in birthing centers—is to eat and drink freely. While the American Society of Anesthesiologists' guidelines from 2007 state that women should avoid solid food, a recent study presented at the society's annual meeting in 2015 showed that women and their babies actually benefit from a light meal during labor. Eating fruit, light soups, a small sandwich, Jell-O, juice, or granola bars provides the energy required for labor. Women who don't eat will burn fat for energy, producing ketones and lactic acid in the same way would someone who is vigorously exercising. As a result, contractions slow down and labor can be extended by forty-five to ninety minutes.

You should not eat during labor if you are at a high risk for aspiration. This includes women who are nauseous, have severe preeclampsia, are obese, or are using opiates for pain relief. If you are unable to eat or drink, you should receive IV fluids (see page 235).

Epidurals

In our culture, pain is viewed as an indication that something is wrong. It is unacceptable and needs to be eliminated. In the case of labor, however, pain is not the sign of something wrong but the sign of something significant happening. About 70 percent of women in the United States who have a vaginal delivery use an epidural during labor. The epidural is the most effective technique for pain relief and is considered the "gold standard."

Injecting anesthesia into a woman's back for childbirth began in the early 1900s. The Swiss obstetrician Dr. Oskar Kreis used cocaine injections to numb his laboring patients completely. In the 1960s, the epidural catheter was developed, allowing the medication to be given continuously throughout labor instead of as a single injection. In the 1980s, anesthesiologists began to add opiates to the local anesthetics so that pain relief was improved.

Currently, most epidurals are actually combination spinal-epidurals, which have a rapid onset of pain relief (within a few minutes) while still allowing the woman to move and feel her legs. They commonly contain bupivacaine, a local anesthetic, and fentanyl, an opiate. Some hospitals also offer patient-controlled epidural analgesia (PCEA), which allows patients to increase the dose of the medication when they are uncomfortable.

If you have decided to use an epidural, you can have it placed whenever you want. An arbitrary amount of cervical dilation is not required because every woman's perception of pain is different. The timing of epidural placement—either early or late in labor—does not affect the cesarean rate. Your doctor may turn off your epidural as you enter the second stage, so you have more sensation to push effectively.

Epidural Light: The Walking Epidural

A walking epidural offers pain relief while maintaining strength and movement. It contains the same amount of opiate as a regular epidural but the level of local anesthetic is lower. Women with this type of epidural hope to be able to walk, go to the bathroom, and have better strength for pushing. However, when a woman is in active labor, the level of pain relief is often inadequate and most will ask for more medication. While they may feel some strength in their legs, it is still difficult to walk. For the hospital, having someone walking while using anesthesia is a significant safety concern. If the woman were to fall, it could be dangerous for her and her baby.

Walking epidurals have been described as the perfect combination of pain relief and retained mobility. However, most women with walking epidurals never walk at all, choosing to sleep and rest instead. Nonetheless, this technique gives women a better perception of their overall birthing experience.

the doctor's diary

I have seen patients who have planned extensively for a natural delivery who eventually opt for an epidural and feel terribly guilty and disappointed, as if they have let someone down. In their childbirth preparation classes, they have been told about risks with epidurals and have convinced themselves that they should never have one. Since you have no idea how long your labor will last and how intense the pain will be, I believe that you should avoid making any specific decisions about pain medication until you have actually felt the pain.

In the end, the majority of patients use epidurals. I have never seen a major complication from one—nobody ends up paralyzed, no babies have permanent damage. I can say with confidence that they are safe. They are just a different way of doing things. Untreated severe pain has potential consequences of its own including failure to progress during labor resulting in a cesarean and postpartum depression.

Benefits of an Epidural

Epidurals grant an essentially pain-free, fully alert labor and birth. For women who have lost the ability to relax due to the intensity and frequency of painful contractions, having an epidural gives a much needed break. This rest period, which may include sleeping, is rejuvenating. For women who are frantic, emotionally overwhelmed, and cannot find relief naturally, an epidural can be a lifesaver, resulting in a positive birth experience. Many women ask for an epidural because they haven't prepared or practiced any pain-relieving techniques, such as hypnobirthing or visualization; they are simply afraid of the pain; or the natural methods haven't worked.

Drawbacks of an Epidural

While great for resolving pain, epidurals lead to a variety of interventions, changes in the labor process, and side effects.

- Inadequate pain relief is seen in 10 percent of patients.
- Fetal heart rate decelerations occur in one third of women with epidurals.
- Most hospitals have protocols that require women with epidurals to have an IV and continuous fetal monitoring.
- Hypotension (low blood pressure) occurs in 80 percent of women with epidurals but can be prevented by giving IV fluids prior to the epidural placement. (This is why all women with epidurals need an IV).
- Without the sensation of contractions to guide them, women cannot change positions to encourage the baby to rotate through its cardinal movements. As a result, more fetuses remain occiput posterior. Without an epidural, 3 percent of babies will stay in the occiput posterior position; with an epidural, 13 percent stay in this position.
- Spinal headaches occur when there is an accidental puncture of the dura, one of the membranes surrounding the spinal cord. Characteristically, this rare complication is only felt when the woman is upright. When lying down, the headache resolves.
- Itching from the opiate component is seen in 58 percent of patients with spinal-epidurals.
- Permanent nerve damage occurs in 1 per 240,000.
- The second stage of labor increases by 1 to 2 hours.
- A woman cannot feel when her bladder is full, so a Foley catheter must be placed to drain the urine.
- Maternal fever occurs in 20 percent of patients and is due to changes in a woman's ability to regulate her temperature.

The fever may prompt an investigation about infection in the newborn, which separates the mother and baby after delivery.

- There is a higher chance that a woman will need to have Pitocin to stimulate stalled labor.
- A spinal-epidural lowers natural oxytocin levels. By numbing the pain, the positive feedback loop that governs the release of oxytocin is disrupted.
- There is an increased use of vacuum and forceps. Six percent of women with epidurals will need an assisted delivery.
- There is an increase in cesarean rates for fetal distress, but no increase in the overall cesarean rate.

Myths About Epidurals

- Epidurals cause back pain: According to many studies, the incidence of back pain after delivery is the same for women who had an epidural and those who didn't.
- Epidurals inhibit mother-newborn bonding: While epidurals lower oxytocin levels, most women who have them are adamant that they bond with their baby just as much.
- Epidurals have long-term effects on the child: No studies clearly indicate an effect on brain development in children.
- Breastfeeding will be more difficult: Some suggest that the narcotics from an epidural make the newborn drowsy and therefore breastfeeding is more difficult. While a small amount of the medication in the epidural gets into the mother's blood stream, she does not get drowsy. Therefore, it is unlikely that the baby is affected in this way. Overall, neurologic exams on newborns are similar for those exposed to epidurals and those who weren't. At this time, there aren't any conclusive studies on the relationship between epidurals and nursing.

Nitrous Oxide

Nitrous oxide is a nonnarcotic, inhaled pain medication, commonly known as laughing gas, which is often used in dentistry. While it does not completely eliminate pain like an epidural, women using nitrous find the pain much more tolerable. Half of laboring women in the United Kingdom, Australia, Canada, and the Netherlands use nitrous oxide. It is currently only available at a few hospitals and birthing centers in the United States, but many are evaluating it as a future option.

The gas is inhaled through a mask as a contraction starts. Peak pain relief takes place in forty-five seconds and wears off in a few minutes. Side effects are mild dizziness and nausea. Women using nitrous can still move around between contractions. Although it crosses the placenta, it does not affect the fetus in any way.

Nitrous oxide may be ideal for women who need pain medication but want to preserve their mobility. It can also be used while awaiting the availability of an anesthesiologist for an epidural, when an epidural is ineffective, or when a woman is too far along (9 to 10 cm dilated) to get an epidural.

the doctor's diary

I have never used nitrous oxide because it isn't available in most hospitals. I have asked my anesthesia colleagues their opinion about its use and they are resistant to it. One asked me, "Why would you recommend it? Don't you like anesthesiologists?" I realized that anesthesiologists may feel threatened by the use of forms of pain relief that don't require them to administer it. Epidurals are their bread and butter, after all. A large hospital in my area had been discussing the viability of using nitrous oxide, but the anesthesia group strongly opposed it, so the idea did not come to fruition.

Narcotics

Narcotics work on the opiate receptors in the brain to dull pain. Those most commonly used in labor are Nubain, Demerol, and

Stadol, given as injections through an IV or directly into muscle. They take effect within minutes and last for two to three hours. Women who are fearful of epidurals often choose narcotics.

Narcotics do not eliminate pain completely but "take the edge off." Once you have taken a narcotic, you cannot walk due its side effects of drowsiness, dizziness, and nausea. Narcotics cross the placenta easily and can make the baby drowsy as well. Effects of narcotics can be seen in a newborn for a few days after delivery. Mothers who receive narcotics within one to three hours of birth usually aren't able to breastfeed effectively until at least twenty hours later.

Electronic Fetal Monitoring

During labor, the uterine muscle contracts so strongly that the blood flow through the uterus temporarily decreases. Most babies adapt to this easily; in fact, they are designed to do so. But some babies can't tolerate it and will drop their heart rate to compensate for the lower oxygen levels. Known as fetal heart rate decelerations, these can be detected on an electronic heart rate monitor. Almost every baby has some decelerations during labor. The question is how many is too many; at what point do the decelerations cause permanent damage, such as cerebral palsy, or even death?

Continuous Fetal Monitoring

Continuous electronic fetal monitoring (CEFM) began in the 1970s. It involves placing two disks on the mother's abdomen and securing them with belts for the duration of labor. One disk is a Doppler ultrasound device, which detects the baby's heart rate. The second measures the pressure generated by uterine contractions.

However, even early on, studies showed that continuous monitoring led to more cesareans but not better outcomes for babies. The incidence of cerebral palsy (2 per 1,000 births) has not changed in the last forty years, despite the use of monitoring, because most cases of cerebral palsy are caused by an incident prior to labor, whereas only 4 percent can be attributed to labor itself.

Although numerous studies showed no benefit, the use of continuous fetal monitoring became widespread. The premature adoption of CEFM has had many consequences: increased cesarean rates, increased use of forceps, increased costs, and legal ramifications. Malpractice lawsuits skyrocketed in the belief that earlier intervention in response to an abnormal fetal heart rate tracing would have improved the outcome. Because the interpretation of the fetal heart rate is largely subjective, even a small deviation from normal, if not acted upon, can be blamed as the cause of a problem with a newborn.

ACOG's guidelines from 2009 say, "Despite the frequency of its use, limitations of electronic fetal monitoring include poor inter-observer reliability, uncertain efficacy, and high false-positive rate"—meaning that different doctors may have different interpretations of the results and that when the heart rate is abnormal, the baby is often perfectly fine. Although intermittent monitoring is an acceptable alternative, 94 percent of women are still monitored continuously.

Risks of Continuous Monitoring
- Increased risk of cesarean by 20 percent
- Increased use of vacuum and forceps
- Highly subjective interpretation of results: Fetal heart rate patterns are not like blood tests, which give a specific numerical result. When four obstetricians were shown a pattern, their interpretation was the same only 22 percent of the time. In addition, when they looked at the same tracings two months later, they changed their diagnosis in 21 percent of the cases.[9]
- Immobility: The belts and cords attached to the monitor allow the mother only a few feet of movement. Wireless fetal monitors that use Wi-Fi or Bluetooth technology are currently being studied but are not yet available in most hospitals.

- Unnecessary stress: CEFM can cause panic in the delivery room. If a baby's heart rate drops, nurses rush into the room from the nursing station where they are monitoring the fetal heart rate remotely. The chaos instills fear in a mother as well as her family. She becomes tense, with her eyes glued to the monitor, afraid for her baby's life. The stress causes the contractions to slow down and she may end up with a cesarean.
- CEFM fosters the unsubstantiated belief that neurologic injury to a baby can always be prevented.

Doctors use CEFM for nearly all laboring women although it hasn't improved outcomes in low-risk patients. Even in the following high-risk situations, there is no data to support its use:

- Fetus with poor growth
- Mothers with preeclampsia or type 1 diabetes
- Women with a prior cesarean
- Women with an infection or fever
- Meconium-stained fluid
- Active vaginal bleeding
- Women receiving Pitocin

Without proof that continuous fetal monitoring is beneficial, why do doctors still prefer it over intermittent monitoring? Mostly because that's what has always been done. Present-day OBs find it challenging to undo forty years of practice and clinical habits. Most doctors and nurses aren't adequately trained in intermittent monitoring and hospitals aren't staffed to accommodate it. Additionally, doctors believe that having a continuous tracing of the heart rate during labor will keep them safe should a problem arise and they are sued. The tracing provides a physical record of labor from beginning to end that can be a key to their defense in a lawsuit.

Intermittent Monitoring

While monitoring the fetus continuously does not improve out-comes, having intermittent monitoring reassures us that the fetus is doing well. Intermittent monitoring protocols state that the provider should listen to the heart rate every fifteen to thirty minutes in active labor and every five to fifteen minutes during pushing. She uses a Doppler device to listen throughout a contraction and for ninety seconds after it ends. If the baby's heart rate is low, it should be monitored again with next contraction. If the rate remains low after two contractions, continuous monitoring should be done.

The problem with intermittent monitoring, and why it is used so infrequently in the United States, is that hospitals aren't adequately staffed to offer it; it requires one-on-one nursing care, which is more expensive and time consuming. One hospital tried to follow the intermittent protocol and was only successful at adhering to the guidelines in 31 of 862 patients. Intermittent monitoring is commonly used in birthing centers and at home.

If your goal is a natural birth, insisting on intermittent fetal monitoring may help you avoid a number of unnecessary interventions. If you are delivering at home or in a birthing center, intermittent monitoring is already the norm. If you are planning a hospital birth, you should talk to your provider about the protocols there. As more women insist on this alternative, rules may finally change and long-standing habits broken.

Vaginal Birth After Cesarean (VBAC)

The debate about how to deliver a baby after a previous cesarean has been going on for one hundred years. "Once a cesarean, always a cesarean" was the mantra of the 1916 meeting of New York ob-gyns. In 1985, 5 percent of women whose previous baby was born via cesarean had a VBAC. As information about the safety of the procedure grew, the rate rose to a high of 28 percent in 1996. However, when

VBACs became more popular, so did the lawsuits, and the rates declined. Currently, only 10 percent of women with a previous cesarean attempt a VBAC. Having a VBAC poses unique risks to the baby. Having a repeat cesarean poses more risk to the mother.

If you previously had a cesarean and want to attempt a vaginal delivery with your next birth, you and your provider need to begin planning for it early in prenatal care. If your first cesarean was scheduled, as in cases of a breech baby or placenta previa, your VBAC success rate is over 80 percent. If the cesarean was because the baby wouldn't come out, the success rate drops to 60 percent. Women who have had a previous vaginal birth, are in spontaneous labor, and are less than forty weeks are more likely to deliver vaginally.

Reasons to Have a VBAC

- Shorter recovery
- Easier to care for newborn and an older child after a vaginal birth
- If you are planning to have more children, multiple cesareans have increased surgical risks.
- Desire to experience a vaginal delivery
- Benefits to the baby of being born vaginally such as seeding its microbiome

Risks of VBAC

- **Uterine rupture:** After a cesarean, a scar forms on the uterus where it was cut. This scar is weaker than normal uterine tissue. When a woman is in labor with a subsequent pregnancy, the strong contractions can cause the scar to open, or rupture. After one cesarean, the risk of uterine rupture is 0.6 percent. After two or more, the risk increases to 1.3 percent. Uterine rupture is more likely if:

○ The previous cesarean occurred less than 18 months ago.
○ You have had two or more cesareans.
○ Your labor has been induced.
○ You had a wound infection after your previous cesarean.
○ You are more than 42 weeks.
○ Your cesarean scar was closed with a single layer of stitches.

The consequences of uterine rupture depend on the time it takes to deliver the baby. In most cases, if the rupture is recognized and the baby delivered within fifteen minutes, the baby will likely be unaffected.

- Fetal distress due to decreased blood flow if a uterine rupture occurs
- Need for hysterectomy because of excessive damage to the uterus
- Fetal injury: Five percent of babies will develop seizures and brain injuries if more than 15 minutes pass from the time of rupture to delivery.
- Fetal death: If more than 30 minutes pass, 65 percent of babies will die. If an emergency cesarean is performed promptly, fetal death occurs in 6 percent. Therefore, with early intervention in a hospital, the risk of fetal death with a VBAC is 0.6 in 1,000, only slightly higher than the chance of a baby's dying during a normal vaginal birth (0.5 in 1,000).

There is no reliable way to predict who will have a complication with a VBAC. Women who shouldn't attempt VBAC are those with:

- A vertical cesarean scar (referring to the scar on the uterus, not on the skin, which is usually done for preemie deliveries)

- A previous uterine rupture
- Two or more previous cesareans
- A placenta previa
- No access to a hospital and anesthesiologist

Risks of Repeat Cesarean

- Injury to surrounding organs, such as the bladder or bowel
- Increased chance of developing a placenta previa or accreta in a subsequent pregnancy
- Longer hospital stay
- The other risks associated with any cesarean, such as pain, infection, and breastfeeding difficulties

Common Hospital Protocols When Attempting VBAC

- A physician and anesthesiologist must be present in the hospital.
- There must be IV access.
- Continuous fetal monitoring should be available.
- Some doctors won't induce patients who want a VBAC because contractions from Pitocin are stronger and more forceful.

the doctor's diary

Half of doctors don't offer VBAC at all; 33 percent of hospitals don't allow them, either. Your provider doesn't get paid for the extra time and effort it takes to monitor a VBAC, nor is there compensation for the additional risk assumed.

The risk of uterine rupture is the number one reason doctors don't support VBACs. In fact, 88 percent of doctors simply recommend a repeat cesarean. From the hospital's perspective, there is little incentive for patients to have a VBAC. The hospital is paid more and incurs less liability with a repeat cesarean.

Women are discouraged in both overt and covert ways from having VBACs. A doctor or nurse may outright say that you are risking the life of your baby, that the outcome can be catastrophic, and that your baby may die. The doctor may also subtly make you question a decision to attempt a VBAC by reiterating at every prenatal appointment that you will need an IV, you will be continuously monitored, and you will need to stay in bed. Since your mobility during labor will be limited, you may question if trying a VBAC is worth it.

I believe that VBACs should be encouraged, as long as they can be done in a safe environment with continuous fetal monitoring and immediate access to an operating room. In this situation, their safety has been well established.

Midwives, Home Birth, and VBAC

If a midwife is working in a hospital, she can offer her patients a VBAC. Some birth centers allow VBACs if the mother meets certain criteria. However, home birth after cesarean (HBAC) is quite controversial. For example, in California, it is illegal for a midwife to attend a VBAC at home. It is still done in some states, however, especially in those where home-birth midwives are not licensed.

A woman who strongly desires a VBAC and can't find a doctor or hospital that will support her doesn't have many options. In fact, it is virtually impossible. Her only choices are to try a home birth or to stay at home as long as possible so that when she arrives at the hospital, she is nearly ready to deliver. Neither of these is a great alternative.

The Midwives Alliance of North America (MANA) studied VBAC at home and found that, while 87 percent of women had a successful VBAC, the chance of fetal death was 2.85 per 1,000, four times higher than a VBAC in the hospital setting (which is 0.6 per 1000).[10]

Please do not attempt a VBAC in your house. If you have a uterine rupture at home—which is a totally unpredictable event—you have less than thirty minutes to recognize it, drive to a hospital, get admitted, have an operating room prepared, and have emergency surgery. Even if your baby survives, it will likely have some degree of injury. I know that an 87 percent success rate sounds good, but the consequences of something going wrong are life-changing.

Unfortunately, many doctors discourage VBAC altogether, even in the hospital setting. This pushes women wanting a VBAC to resort to homebirth or to feel disappointment about a repeat cesarean. Training residents in the numerous benefits of VBAC and encouraging hospitals to offer them again would help women have a safe place to undertake it. Ultimately, the best way to avoid the issue of VBAC is to decrease the rate of cesareans in the first place.

Episiotomy

The vagina is designed to accommodate the birth of a baby. Its folded ridges, called rugae, expand dramatically like an accordion. The perineum, the area between the vagina and anus, also can stretch, as long as the delivery is unrushed.

An episiotomy, first described in 1742, is a cut (incision) made in the perineum as the baby's head is crowning to create more space. It is repaired with stitches after the delivery of the baby and the placenta. Most episiotomies heal within a week or two. They became the standard of care in the 1920s as prominent obstetricians claimed that they would make the perineum stronger, prevent prolapse, and restore virginal conditions after delivery. Episiotomies were routinely done in the 1940s and 1950s because nearly all women were unconscious during labor and doctors used forceps to deliver the baby. Repairing a single episiotomy was easier than multiple, irregular lacerations that occurred with the use of forceps.

Studies in the 1980s showed the opposite of what doctors believed to be true: episiotomies do not prevent prolapse, make the delivery easier, or heal better than lacerations. In fact, they actually cause more damage to the surrounding tissue. When the perineum is intact, it will gradually stretch. But if the perineum has a small cut in it, it will tear even further. Therefore, in 2006, ACOG issued guidelines restricting the use of episiotomy to emergency situations, citing no benefit to their routine use. Today, they are used in 10 percent of deliveries. However, in some hospitals, the episiotomy rate remains high, at 35 percent. Doctors use them to expedite a delivery, especially if they are busy with other patients, or they do them out of habit. Midwives, on the contrary, are trained to deliver keeping the woman's perineum intact, and perform episiotomies in only 1 percent of births.

Vaginal Lacerations

A vaginal laceration is a spontaneous tear in the labia, perineum, or near the urethra. When it occurs inside the walls of the vaginal canal, it is called a sulcal tear. Most lacerations are small and easily repaired. However, some, especially sulcal tears, can bleed excessively so that a woman may require a transfusion. Lacerations occur in the deliveries of 55 percent of first time moms and in 30 percent of those who have given birth before. Midwives take pride in delivering without a vaginal laceration, considering it a badge of honor.

Consequences of Episiotomy

- Episiotomies are more likely to extend to the rectum than a laceration.
- If a woman has an episiotomy with her first delivery, she is 4 times more likely to tear with her second baby because the perineum is permanently weakened.

- Perineal pain is more pronounced.
- Sex can be painful for mothers after delivery.

Preventing Lacerations and the Need for Episiotomies

- Perineal massage during pregnancy can help prepare the birth canal by making the perineum more flexible, decreasing its chance of tearing. You can massage the perineum daily, starting at 34 weeks, with a water-soluble lubricant or natural oils, such as almond or vitamin E oil. (See page 47, on how to prepare your body for birth.)
- A perineal dilator is a balloon that is placed into the vaginal opening and inflated. This can be done during pregnancy, like the perineal massage.
- Hands and knees or side positioning during labor and delivery can reduce the amount of tearing.
- Labor in a water bath allows the muscles to relax.
- Warm compresses applied to the area during the pushing stage of labor can help. The doctor or midwife will wet a washcloth with hot water and lay it on the perineum.
- Delivering with the legs relaxed and not pulled back decreases the tension on the perineum.
- While your natural instinct is to push as hard as possible when the baby is crowning, you are less likely to tear if you breathe deeply and allow the skin time to stretch.
- The doctor or midwife maintains slow, controlled birth of the fetal head in the flexed position. The provider will apply pressure against the head slightly downward, so the head stays flexed as it comes out. If the pressure isn't applied, the head can snap back as it comes through the opening and tear the skin.

the doctor's diary

Perineal massage by your doctor while you are pushing was believed to reduce tearing and the need for episiotomy. However, constantly rubbing the perineum only makes the tissue sore, swollen, and more likely to tear. As one of my favorite midwives described, "How would it feel if you rubbed your fingers against the inside of your mouth for an hour or two? That's how your vagina feels with prolonged perineal massage."

Group B Streptococcus (GBS) Treatment

As discussed on page 139, Group B streptococcus (GBS) is found in 20 to 30 percent of women's genital tracts. It doesn't cause any symptoms in mothers, but can lead to pneumonia, meningitis, and even death in a newborn. Symptoms in the newborn are lethargy, difficulty breathing or feeding, and fevers.

All pregnant women should be screened for GBS between thirty-five and thirty-seven weeks. If a woman tests positive, she should receive antibiotics during labor. At least two doses of antibiotics is given through an IV, four hours apart. Oral and intramuscular injections of antibiotics do not effectively eliminate GBS because they don't reach high enough levels in the uterus. Women who are delivering by cesarean whose water hasn't broken do not need this treatment, though some doctors give it anyway.

Without treatment during labor, 50 percent of babies born to women with GBS will carry the bacteria. Of those, 1 to 2 percent will become infected and 5 percent with an infection will die. Infections in the newborn can occur early, within the first week of life, or late, between two to twelve weeks. Treatment during labor is specifically to prevent early-onset disease. There is no way to prevent the late-onset form.

Amniotomy should be avoided for GBS carriers, or at least postponed until antibiotics have been given. If the water bag breaks on its own during labor, cervical exams should be kept to a minimum to decrease the risk of pushing the bacteria into the uterus.

Chlorhexidine, an antiseptic cleansing solution, can be applied to the vaginal canal or used to clean the newborn after delivery to decrease the risk of GBS infections. This cleanser is beneficial for women giving birth in developing countries where antibiotics are not readily available. It should not be considered an alternative to antibiotics.

Other approaches to eliminating GBS from the genital tract include garlic and lactobacillus. While a few studies show promise, there is not yet definitive evidence that these methods work in humans. The future of GBS prevention will likely involve a vaccine.

Women who are GBS positive and want to have a natural birth can do so. In a hospital, birthing center or even at home, a saline lock can be placed and IV antibiotics given every four hours. The medicine runs through the IV in fifteen minutes, after which the tubing can be disconnected. Licensed midwives are able to administer these antibiotics in the home.

To minimize your risk of carrying GBS, you can use a probiotic such as lactobacillus during pregnancy. While studies on this option are limited, there may be some benefit. However, you should still be screened. Don't try to trick the test by retesting if you've had a positive result. While GBS may come and go, if you have ever tested positive, you should be treated as such. In labor, ask your provider to minimize cervical exams and avoid artificial rupture of membranes.

Assisted Deliveries

Assisted deliveries are done if a mother cannot push the baby out or if the baby's heart rate drops, necessitating an urgent delivery. Unfortunately, they are also performed because the doctor is impatient or in a rush. Just over 4 percent of deliveries in the United States are done with a device to pull the baby out, such as forceps or a vacuum. Forceps look like two oversized salad spoons joined together at their handles. A vacuum is a small plastic cup that fits on the baby's head and that attaches to a handheld suction pump via a long tube.

Assisted deliveries were first described during the Middle Ages. Kitchen utensils were used to save the life of the mother and to assist in deliveries that were prolonged and lasted many days. In the early 1900s, over 60 percent of deliveries in the United States were done with forceps.

These deliveries should only be attempted if the cervix is fully dilated, the fetal head is low, and the baby is not excessively large. The doctor's decision whether to use a vacuum or forceps depends on her training and expertise.

Complications of Assisted Deliveries

Trauma to the baby: Although rare, bleeding in the brain, bruises and cuts on the face, and skull fractures can occur.

Maternal complications: Deep lacerations to the birth canal, future urinary incontinence, or painful intercourse.

The best way to avoid needing an assisted delivery is to optimize your ability to push the baby out:

- Avoid epidurals. Because epidurals can limit your strength, they increase the need for forceps and vacuum by 40 percent.
- Let the baby labor down.
- Push instinctively when you feel the greatest urge at the peak of a contraction.
- Hire a doula who can help you with varied positions during labor and effective pushing techniques.
- Use upright or side positions during pushing.

Finding the Balance

Numerous technologies and advances in medicine have transformed childbirth from a risky proposition one hundred years ago to an event in which we can almost always count on a positive outcome. There is no doubt that these advances have also "medicalized" birth. I am always disappointed to hear of patients who felt that they had things done to them without even knowing why. But then I think of my own first pregnancy. Without significant medical intervention, I would not be here today. Severe preeclampsia led to an induction with Pitocin, staying in bed, hooked to an IV, continuous fetal monitoring, an epidural, and ultimately the birth of my son at thirty-one weeks. I could not be more grateful to have had these options.

Having a cesarean for a placenta previa is an example of a life-saving intervention, whereas having a episiotomy because it is the habit of your doctor can be harmful. Even a seemingly insignificant intervention, such as having an IV, can lead to a cascade of further interventions: immobility leads to an epidural that causes a drop in maternal blood pressure that triggers a fetal heart rate deceleration that culminates in an emergency cesarean. Finding a balance between the natural and the medicalized is our greatest challenge in modern obstetrics.

Here's a summary of things that are commonly done during low-risk pregnancies and labor that haven't been scientifically proven to benefit you or your baby:

- Ultrasound
- Prenatal vitamins
- Nonstress tests and biophysical profiles
- Amniotic fluid evaluation
- Bed rest
- Continuous fetal monitoring in labor

- Breaking the water bag during labor
- Adhering strictly to Friedman's labor curve
- Having an IV during labor
- Prohibiting eating and drinking during labor
- Labor induction for big babies, low amniotic fluid, or passing the due date

Questions to Ask Your Doctor or Midwife About Labor

- What is your cesarean rate?
- How far past my due date can I go?
- Can I await spontaneous labor?
- Can I wait for my water to break on its own?
- Can I have intermittent monitoring?
- Can you minimize cervical exams?
- Do I have to have an IV? Can I eat during labor?
- What options are available for pain relief? Are there birthing tubs? Do you offer nitrous oxide or TENS units? Does the hospital offer walking epidurals?
- Can I stay mobile during labor?
- Can I delay pushing until I have the urge?
- Can I push in any position?
- Can I wait to clamp and cut the cord?
- If I have had a cesarean in the past, do you allow VBAC?

THE UNPREDICTABLE, WONDERFUL, VERY SPECIAL DAY

S OME PREGNANCIES ARE HIGH RISK BEFORE THEY BEGIN. OTHERS develop problems during the forty weeks. But if you've made it through the pregnancy with no complications, you may assume that your birth will be simple. After all, once you're in labor, it's just another twenty-four hours or so. But, believe it or not, 30 percent of women with no risk factors at all have a complication during labor or delivery, or an issue with their newborn right after birth.

Just as it is important to plan for how you would like your labor and delivery to be, it is important to understand the circumstances that could require those plans to change. These include infections during labor, unexpected cesareans, and meconium passage. The more you know about the possibilities, the better equipped you will be to prevent them or cope with them effectively.

Delivery in the Hospital

You have been admitted to the hospital in labor and set up a comfortable place for yourself in the delivery room. You have your pillow, music, and a birthing ball. Your support team is standing by. Childbirth classes have explained what to expect from here. You are as ready as you can be.

You will notice that there are a lot of beeping machines in your room. Your IV sounds an alarm if its tubing gets kinked. The fetal heart rate monitor beeps if the baby's heart rate goes below a certain level. The blood pressure machine alarm will go off if the reading is too high.

You overhear your nurse quietly calling your doctor. "She's febrile. Her cervix is edematous. The baby has mec and she's having decels." You are not sure what it means, but it doesn't sound good. Deciphering the medical jargon can be a challenge in itself, especially while in labor.

A number of common conditions and situations may develop during your labor and delivery. Some impact you and others concern your baby. The following will help you understand what can happen and how certain situations are treated. Remember that if your doctor or nurse uses terminology you do not understand, don't hesitate to ask what it means.

Fever

A fever is a maternal temperature of 100.4 degrees Fahrenheit or higher. Fevers during labor may result from infections but can also arise from other causes. A woman can develop a fever simply from laboring in an overheated room. In addition, 20 percent of women with an epidural will develop a fever within one to four hours of its placement. Women who are obese as well as those with prolonged labors are also more likely to develop a fever.

LABOR AND DELIVERY LINGO

When you are in labor, your doctors and nurses may seem to be speaking a different language. The following are some of the common terms and phrases that you may hear in the delivery or operating room.

She's a prime. = It's her first baby.

She's a multip. = She's had a baby before.

I need to check you now. = I will do a cervical exam to see how dilated you are.

I'm going to rupture you now. = I'm going to break your water bag.

She's complete. = She is 10 cm dilated and 100 percent effaced.

We need to Pit her out. = She needs to be induced with Pitocin.

She has a lip. = The cervix is swollen in the front.

She needs a whiff of Pit. = The contractions have slowed and she needs Pitocin to make them stronger.

Let it labor down. = When a woman is completely dilated but doesn't have the urge to push, she can allow the uterus to push the baby through the birth canal without maternal effort.

She's minus two. = The baby's head is high.

She's febrile. = She has a fever.

The baby is OP./The baby is sunny-side up. = The fetal head is rotated so that the back of the baby's head is near the mother's spine.

She has oligo. = The fluid around the baby is low.

She has mec./It's pea soup. = The amniotic fluid is green because the baby has passed meconium.

She's a VBAC. = She wants to have a vaginal delivery after a previous cesarean delivery.

She's having decels. = The baby's heart rate has dropped.

She's SROM-NIL. = Her water has broken but she isn't having any contractions.

She's arrested. = She isn't making any progress in labor.

I have to cut her. = She needs a cesarean.

I'm taking her to the back. = The nurse is moving the patient to the operating room for a cesarean.

We need to crash her. = She needs an emergency cesarean NOW.

Eyes and thighs = The antibiotic eye ointment and the vitamin K injection, which are routinely given to babies after birth

Fevers are concerning because they may be a sign of chorio-amnionitis, an infection within the uterus caused by bacteria from the vaginal canal. Once the amniotic sac is broken, these bacteria migrate into the uterus. If the bag of water has been broken for a prolonged period of time or if the mother has had multiple cervical exams, she is more likely to develop this condition. Because chorio-amnionitis can cause severe infections in the baby, a mother with a fever will be treated with IV antibiotics. If she is in the early stages of labor and delivery is not imminent, many doctors will recommend a cesarean.

A Swollen Cervix

The cervix opens in the shape of an oval during early labor, and forms a circle in the later stages. Simultaneously, the cervix thins, or effaces. If the fetal head presses too hard against the cervix, the blood flow through the cervical tissue is limited, the cervix swells, and dilation stops. A swollen cervix is a common cause of a cesarean.

The cervix swells if the woman is involuntarily pushing down against a cervix that isn't fully dilated, but more often it occurs because the baby's head is positioned so that the blood can't circulate normally. Because the cervix dilates as an oval, cervical swelling is often asymmetric. An "anterior lip" develops when the cervix swells only in the front of the baby's head.

The best way to correct a swollen cervix is to change positions—especially hands-and-knees. Once the baby's head moves, normal circulation is restored and the swelling goes down. If the cervix is swollen only on one side, you should lie on the opposite side to relieve the pressure. Resting in a quiet room or birthing tub may alleviate swelling by allowing relaxation of the pelvic muscles.

Some midwives advocate putting ice in a sterile glove inside the vagina against the cervix. Evening primrose oil and homeopathic tablets of arnica have also been suggested as remedies. However, evidence on these strategies is anecdotal only. In some cases, your provider can push the swollen cervix around the baby's head during a contraction, rendering the cervix completely dilated.

Meconium

Meconium is the first stool of a newborn. Normally, meconium is passed in the first day after birth. However, 10 percent of the time, a fetus passes meconium prior to delivery. The diagnosis of meconium can only be made after the amniotic sac has broken. Normal amniotic fluid is clear or pale yellow, but fluid containing meconium will have a dark green or brown color.

Meconium is more common as a woman goes beyond her due date. At forty-two weeks, 17 percent of babies will have passed meconium. It happens because the gastrointestinal tract is ready to begin normal function; it can also occur as a reaction to stress before and during labor. It is impossible to know exactly why a baby passed its meconium, so it isn't reliable as an indicator of fetal distress.

Most babies who pass meconium have no problems, but 2 percent will develop meconium aspiration syndrome (MAS) in which the baby draws the meconium into its lungs with its first few breaths. Fetal distress during labor causes a baby to gasp at birth, increasing the chance of MAS. Meconium in the lungs causes breathing difficulties by blocking the airways and causing inflammation or infection. Three percent of babies with MAS will die.

Meconium passage leads to many other interventions. Although it would seem logical to keep a fetus that has passed meconium from becoming stressed so that it doesn't gasp at birth, common practices actually achieve the opposite effect. Most hospital policies insist on continuous fetal monitoring when meconium is present. This leads to bed rest, needing an epidural, Pitocin use, and a higher chance for a cesarean. Staff from the NICU will usually attend the birth of babies who have passed meconium to evaluate for aspiration.

If you are attempting a home birth, you should transfer to a hospital if the meconium is thick. If delivery is imminent when you discover the meconium, you should bring the baby to the hospital for evaluation after birth.

To decrease the risk of MAS:

- Wait for spontaneous labor.
- Push instinctively.
- Create a relaxing birth environment.

Nonreassuring Fetal Status (a.k.a. Fetal Distress)

Monitoring the fetal heart rate during labor is done for nearly all pregnant women either intermittently or continuously. The goal of monitoring is to identify heart rate patterns that are dangerous to the fetus and to intervene early to prevent problems such as cerebral palsy, brain damage, or stillbirth. However, as previously discussed, continuous fetal monitoring has never been proven to reduce the incidence of these problems. The heart rate patterns are a poor predictor of the baby's health in the short and long term. Abnormal heart rate patterns are responsible for one quarter of cesareans. Despite our attempts to classify the changes in fetal heart rate and to create guidelines for management, interpretation is largely subjective. Ultimately, it is a judgment call that will be made by your doctor.

Variable Decelerations

A variable deceleration is a sudden drop in the fetal heart rate during a contraction that returns to normal when the contraction finishes. This characteristic pattern is caused by a pinched umbilical cord, which occurs when the cord is around the baby's neck or between the baby's body and the uterine wall. It is more common when the amniotic fluid is low.

Changing positions allows the cord to fall into a different place. However, when delivering in a hospital, variables often initiate protocols that require a woman to get an IV and stay in bed with the continuous fetal monitor, which may be the exact opposite of what she needs.

Amnioinfusion is a treatment for recurrent variable decelerations. Your provider will place an intrauterine pressure catheter (IUPC)—a flexible plastic tube—into the uterus. Sterile water is then infused into the uterus to give the umbilical cord a cushion. Studies have shown that amnioinfusion reduces the occurrence of variables, and therefore decreases the cesarean rate.

Variable decelerations are common, and babies are rarely affected unless they occur with nearly all contractions. However, because there is no specific number of variables that indicate danger, frequent variables often prompt a cesarean.

Late Decelerations

With each contraction, uterine blood vessels are squeezed and the blood flow slows temporarily. As a result, the oxygen supply to the baby also declines. The natural breaks between contractions allow the blood supply to resume. If the baby cannot tolerate the lower oxygen levels, its heart rate will slow. This pattern, a drop in the heart rate starting at the peak of a contraction and continuing after the contraction has ended, is known as a late deceleration. Late decelerations that occur with more than half of the contractions are associated with fetal brain damage and stillbirth. However, as with variables, there is no exact number that is known to be harmful.

Medical treatment for late decelerations involves giving oxygen to the mother, administering IV fluids, positioning the mother on her side, and giving medication to temporarily stop contractions. If these techniques do not work, a cesarean will be done.

Early Decelerations

An early deceleration is a drop in the fetal heart rate that mirrors a contraction. It starts at the beginning of the contraction and returns to normal at the end of the contraction. Early decelerations are a reaction to pressure on the baby's head within the birth canal. They are not dangerous and are often seen when labor is progressing quickly.

Preventing Fetal Distress

- Allow labor to start spontaneously.
- Avoid unnecessary inductions.
- Be patient during labor to avoid the use of Pitocin.
- Move around frequently and change positions.
- Stay well hydrated by drinking lots of water and eating small amounts of food, especially during early labor unless you have a condition that precludes eating during labor.
- Don't lie flat on your back, which can lower blood pressure.
- Allow the water to break on its own.
- Ask your provider whether you can have your baby monitored intermittently so that you can move around freely.

Nuchal Cord

Nuchal cord is the term used when the umbilical cord is wrapped around a baby's neck, a concept that instills fear in many women. The potential concern about nuchal cords is not that the baby can't breathe, but that the blood flow through the cord would cease. One in three babies are born with a nuchal cord. As the baby moves, the cord wraps around the neck, forming one or more loops that can be loose or tight and even tie a complete knot.

Nuchal cords are rarely dangerous for the baby. There are three umbilical blood vessels—two arteries and a vein—that are protected within the cord by a thick substance called Wharton's jelly. The gel cushions the vessels from serious damage.

Nuchal cords can sometimes be identified on an ultrasound during pregnancy. Detecting a cord around the neck, especially early on, does not mean it will stay that way. In fact, over 75 percent of nuchal cords seen at thirty weeks had resolved by thirty-eight weeks. Some doctors, and patients, want to deliver by cesarean if a nuchal cord is seen on the ultrasound, but there is no evidence to support this practice.

Because nuchal cords are a common reason for variable decelerations, they are the cause for many cesareans. However, when there are no signs of fetal distress, a baby can be born vaginally with a nuchal cord. Most cords are loose and can be easily unwrapped once the baby's head has delivered. The baby can also be delivered with the cord still around its neck. However, occasionally, the cord tightens as the head emerges. In these cases, the cord will need to be clamped and cut so that the baby can be delivered.

Arrest of Dilation

Arrest of dilation means that the active phase of labor has slowed or stopped. Also known as failure to progress, it is the most common reason for unplanned cesareans. The original description of normal labor by Dr. Emanuel Friedman in the 1950s suggested that the cervix should dilate at least 1.2 cm per hour. When labor falls outside of this range, a cesarean is recommended. Dr. Friedman's original labor curve may not be applicable today, though, as labors generally take longer than they did sixty years ago. If modern labors are compared to the Friedman curve, almost 40 percent will be "abnormal."

Arrest of dilation can only be diagnosed in the active phase. Dr. Friedman originally designated 4 cm as the point of transition from the latent to active phase. However, more recent data suggest that active labor begins at 6 cm. Although the accepted definition of active labor has changed, half of women who have a cesarean for "arrest of dilation" do so before they reach 5 cm and aren't truly in active labor.

Doctors adhere to the Friedman curve because they assume that slow progress is a sign that the baby doesn't "fit" and that it may get stuck on its way out, resulting in a shoulder dystocia. When a lawsuit results from shoulder dystocia, the prosecution is quick to question the labor curve. If the patient's labor didn't follow Friedman's curve exactly, lawyers will suggest that the doctor could have prevented the shoulder dystocia by performing a cesarean. However, in most cases, a slow labor is not dangerous for mother or baby.

Cervical dilation may slow due to:

- Uterine hypocontractility: The uterine contractions are not strong enough to dilate the cervix.
- Obesity: The active phase averages two hours longer in obese women.
- Cephalopelvic disproportion (CPD): The baby's head (cephalo) is too big for its mother's pelvis. CPD has less to do with the actual size of the baby's head and more to do with the angle that the head takes as it navigates the birth canal. Rotation of the baby's head occurs spontaneously, and happens more easily when the mother is allowed to move around and change positions regularly. Many babies that are "stuck" or "too big" just need more time to complete the cardinal movements of labor. CPD cannot accurately be predicted because the precise size of your pelvis and the baby are not known. Nonetheless, many doctors suggest having a cesarean for this reason before labor has even started.
- Being confined to bed: By moving around, her pelvis shifts so that the baby can fit through the birth canal easier.
- Being older: Older mothers have longer labors.
- Having your first baby: First babies take twice as long as second babies.
- Stress/fear: Labor slows due to stress and fear. Arriving in an unfamiliar hospital setting and having interventions during labor causes stress hormones to rise and oxytocin to fall.

How to Encourage Dilation

There are natural and medical options that can be pursued when dilation stalls.

- Master relaxation techniques during pregnancy. You should think about what helps you to feel relaxed and peaceful. Is it visualization? Is it hypnosis? Practice these techniques often so that they will be second nature while you are in labor.
- Discover whether you have any fears or negative connotations about childbirth. Your preconceived ideas may hold you back from relaxing fully. Working with a doula during pregnancy can help you uncover these issues and resolve them.
- Find a provider who supports the idea that labor takes time. If your doctor adheres strictly to the Friedman curve, you may want to consider switching your care to someone else. Midwives are generally more flexible about these guidelines.
- Be patient: Labor does not need to follow a strict timeline. If you are less than 6 cm dilated, you are not yet in active labor. Allowing time to pass so that your body can progress to the next phase of labor will lower the chances of a diagnosis of arrest of dilation.
- Create a peaceful environment with soft lights, a warm room, and music. This can be done in any birth setting, even a hospital. You can ask to have the lights dimmed or turned off. Flameless candles, incense, or diffusers with scented oils create a serene mood. Bring a portable speaker to play music. Ask your nurse to turn up the thermostat if the room is chilly. Bring along your own comfortable blankets and pillows.

- Labor in a warm shower or bath.
- Invite people to attend your labor who will keep up your morale if labor is long.
- Walk: Walking and changing position may help the baby rotate so that cervical dilation may resume.
- Increase oral or IV intake of fluids: The uterine muscle will contract more effectively when you are well hydrated.
- Avoid looking at the clock or calculating how long you have been in labor. When you feel pressured to deliver by a certain time or when you feel discouraged that your labor is taking too long, you may find it harder to relax.
- Pitocin: Pitocin is an IV medication used to increase the strength and frequency of uterine contractions. The use of Pitocin in this situation is called labor augmentation.
- Amniotomy: Breaking the water bag is commonly done for women with slow labor, though it is not always effective.
- Epidural: While an epidural may slow some labors, it helps other women to relax so progress may resume. If natural methods of pain relief haven't been effective and a mother is suffering, an epidural can be the perfect solution to relieve her tense muscles.

Arrest of Descent

Arrest of descent is diagnosed when the baby won't come out despite adequate pushing for three and a half hours for a first-time mom with an epidural, and three hours without an epidural. Even with these accepted guidelines, one third of women who have a cesarean for arrest of descent haven't pushed for the designated amount of time.

Pushing for a long time can lead to bleeding excessively after delivery (postpartum hemorrhage) or developing a uterine infection. Prolonged periods of pushing do not, however, affect the baby.

Causes of arrest of descent include:

- Occiput posterior position (OP): If the baby is OP, the second stage of labor is 50 percent longer.
- Epidural: Epidurals prolong the second stage of labor by one to two hours because they numb the sensation to push.
- Stress: Similar to an arrest of dilation, stress triggers hormones that slow contractions.
- Big baby: The baby simply won't fit because it is too big for the mother's pelvis.

Helping Resolve Arrested Descent

- Move around frequently: This will encourage the proper rotation of the baby's head. Pushing in different positions, especially lying on the side or being on hands and knees, will give the baby extra space. Sitting upright and squatting utilizes the force of gravity.
- Empty your bladder: A full bladder can block the path of the baby.
- Use natural techniques for pain relief during labor: Having an epidural increases the chance that the baby will remain in the occiput posterior position and blunts your urge to push.
- Push instinctively: By allowing the contraction to guide you, you conserve energy. Pushing as the contraction peaks is more effective than pushing as soon as it starts. (See page 205, on pushing patterns.)
- Allow delayed pushing: Uterine contractions alone push the baby through the birth canal. When you wait to push until you have a strong urge, the risk of arrest of descent and need for cesarean decreases.
- Have an assisted delivery: Have your doctor use a vacuum to pull the baby out.
- Turn down the epidural: When the epidural is at full strength, pushing will be challenging because you cannot

feel your contractions. Turning down the epidural, or shutting it off completely, allows you to regain normal sensation within thirty to ninety minutes. Once you are not as numb, you will know when the contractions are happening and be able to coordinate your muscles for more effective pushing.

Making it all the way to the pushing phase and not being able to deliver the baby is incredibly discouraging. Sometimes, a doctor or nurse will imply (or even say directly) that you're not trying hard enough, which is clearly not the case. Having a cesarean in this situation is also physically challenging. Not only have you been through an entire labor, but now you are having major surgery. Arrest of descent, of all the reasons for cesareans, results in the most difficult recovery.

The diagnosis of both arrest disorders—arrest of dilation and arrest of descent—is also influenced by factors unrelated to you. Having a limited number of delivery rooms that require one patient to deliver so another can use the room may motivate hospital staff to expedite a delivery. Doctors' fatigue or other duties in the office prompt physicians to say that labor has stalled so they can complete the delivery and move on to the next patient. If your doctor recommends that you need a cesarean for an arrest disorder, you can ask him whether it is safe to try a little longer. Make sure that all of your options have been tried, like changing positions or resting for a while to restore your energy.

Water Has Broken but Contractions Haven't Begun

Most labors begin with contractions, but for 10 to 15 percent of women, the water breaks first. Half of women will go into labor within twelve hours thereafter, and 95 percent will go into labor within twenty-four hours. But what if you are in that 5 percent who don't go into labor after your water breaks?

When 24 hours have passed since the water has broken and contractions have not started spontaneously, the standard approach is to induce labor. The idea of being "on the clock" began in the 1960s, when stillbirth rates for women who had not gone into labor after the water broke were very high. Many of these women had no prenatal care at all, didn't receive antibiotics until infections were severe, and weren't offered timely cesarean sections.

Women who are more likely to break their water bag and not go into labor are those with vaginal infections during pregnancy—such as yeast or bacterial vaginosis—and those who received weekly cervical exams in the last month.

While the greatest concern about prolonged rupture of membranes is an infection in the newborn, labor induction has not been shown to decrease that risk. Inducing does, however, slightly decrease the risk of infection in the mother especially if she doesn't have many cervical exams.[1] Immediate induction and waiting for labor are both reasonable options.[2]

If your water breaks and you aren't in labor, the most important thing you can do is avoid multiple cervical exams. You should continue to walk and move around frequently. Nipple stimulation can also be tried to encourage contractions.

Occiput Posterior

Occiput posterior (OP) is a fetal position in which the back of the baby's head is near the mother's spine. When a baby is OP, its neck is extended and it is unable to tuck its chin. Therefore, the diameter of the head that needs to fit through the birth canal is wider, and vaginal delivery is more difficult. This position is also called sunny-side up because a baby will come out with its eyes looking toward the ceiling like two eggs on a plate.

The best way to determine whether a baby is OP is an ultrasound. Cervical exams early in labor and feeling the mother's abdomen are not as accurate. Once the cervix is sufficiently dilated, your provider can feel for the fontanel (soft spot) on the baby's skull to confirm the diagnosis.

A baby enters the pelvis, the pelvic inlet, with its head sideways so that it is facing one of its mother's hips. Normally, it rotates so that the back of the head, the largest part, sits in front, near the mother's pubic bone. If it instead rotates the opposite direction, the baby will be OP.

Although many babies (25 percent) start labor OP, 95 percent will naturally rotate during labor so they deliver in the occiput anterior (OA) position. If a baby remains OP, arrests of dilation and descent are more common. The chance of a cesarean is four to ten times higher and the second stage of labor increases by 50 percent.

Babies are more likely to be OP if:

- The mother has an epidural.
- The mother is obese.
- The baby is large.
- The placenta is anterior (on the front wall of the uterus).
- The pelvis is narrow.
- The mother is having her first baby.

Myth: If you have back labor, it means your baby is OP. Although this is a common myth, there is no evidence to support it. Just as many women with OA babies have back labor as do women with OP babies. Back labor is caused by tight ligaments and muscles in the pelvis. As the muscles stretch, they pull on the sacrum, causing pain. Walking, sitting on a birthing ball, and applying counterpressure can be helpful to relieve this pain.

Helping a Baby to Rotate

Prior to labor, there is no way to prevent a baby from being OP. If OP is suspected during labor, sitting in a knees-to-chest position will open the pelvis widely, so the baby can rotate. To get in this position, sit on your knees on a padded surface with your hips wide apart. Extend your chest forward, resting it on a large pillow or birthing ball. If you have an epidural and can't balance on your knees, you can lie on your side with your upper leg resting on a stack of pillows. You should allow the bag of water to rupture on its own, maintaining the cushion around the baby as long as possible.

You can also do an abdominal lift to elevate the baby from its stuck position. To do this maneuver, stand with your lower back flat against a wall. Interlock your fingers below your belly. With each contraction, lift your belly 2 to 3 inches upward. When the contraction is done, release your belly. Repeat this ten times.

If your baby still won't turn, your provider can attempt a manual rotation. He will place his hand on the baby's head, flex and rotate it to one side or the other. If manual rotation is attempted before the baby's head is significantly low in the birth canal, it has a 90 percent success rate.

Most women enter labor with a general idea of how it will unfold. But they usually aren't thinking that their baby will have meconium or that their cervix won't dilate past 7 cm. Whatever scenario you are handed, it's unlikely that it's exactly what you envisioned. Accepting these surprises and moving through them with resilience is great practice for parenting. The way you feel when you meet your baby—your confidence and flexibility—will set the tone for your future as a mother. Having a healthy baby is priority number one; embracing the unpredictability of this process so that you can move into motherhood is the next step.

AFTER DELIVERY

MANY PREGNANT WOMEN SPEND A GOOD PORTION OF THE FORTY weeks thinking about and planning their birth but don't consider much beyond their desire for a safe delivery and a healthy baby. If you are like them, you have probably spent lots of time preparing by reading, talking to friends and family, taking childbirth classes, and doing research on the Internet about labor and delivery. You may not have invested as much time figuring out what is going to happen during the hours, weeks, and months after the birth. The postpartum transition is challenging. Days go by without sleep, except for a few hours here and there. Breastfeeding may be harder than you thought it would be. Having a shower in the morning, or even before dinner, is rare. You may not feel close to the baby or your partner.

Visits with your provider are less frequent. At the end of pregnancy, you see your doctor or midwife once or even twice a week. After delivery, you may not see your provider again for six weeks. You may feel alone and unguided. But there are many places to look for help—your pediatrician, your mother, friends from your birthing class, and mommy blogs that you can read in the middle of the night.

Your birth was probably full of surprises. Believe it or not, that was just the beginning of your unpredictable ride. Babies don't come with instruction manuals, and as you journey through this intense, miraculous, and exhausting time, try to remember that every new mom has been in this place, overwhelmed by responsibilities and expectations. You may be inundated with advice from friends and family—sometimes unsolicited or inappropriate. Remember that they are just trying to help, so take the advice in the spirit in which it is given and use what works for you. Every baby is different. You may feel lost; you may feel inadequate. But you may also find yourself filled with confidence and joy as you discover what works best for you and your family. Before you know it, you'll be the most expert parent for your child that there could ever be.

In the Delivery Room and Beyond

After the baby is born, you will spend a few hours recovering in the delivery room. If you had a cesarean, you will be moved from the operating room to a recovery area. If you delivered in a birthing center, you will stay there for about six hours and then go home.

The Baby After Birth

Initially, a baby will cry because it is suddenly exposed to the unfamiliar sensation of being in the outside world. The cry works to expand its lungs and expel mucus and amniotic fluid. Following a short stage of quiet relaxation, lasting a few minutes, the baby will rouse itself and make intentional movements toward the breast, guided by the sound of its mother's voice and the smell of her body. A baby lying on its mother's abdomen, skin to skin, will move on its own to the breast, a phenomenon called the breast crawl. Of course,

YOUR BABY'S MICROBIOME

Nearly 75 percent of our immune cells are found within the intestinal tract, where our body is first exposed to toxins and infections. The "good" bacteria that live here play a major role in triggering immune cells to produce antibodies that fight disease. They also stop the immune system from overreacting to nonharmful substances, which is how allergies develop.

The microbiome consists of the variety of organisms, such as yeast and bacteria, which live within the human body. When a baby is born, its intestinal tract is essentially sterile with very few bacteria present. Populating the intestines with good bacteria is essential to the health of the newborn, and will also prevent disease through childhood and adulthood.

You help to establish the microbiome of your baby in three ways:

1. Your vaginal bacteria cover the baby during childbirth.
2. Bacteria from your skin coat the skin, nose, and mouth of the baby.
3. Your breast milk contains over 700 species of bacteria.

To ensure that your baby develops a healthy microbiome:

- Avoid douching during pregnancy. Douching unnecessarily eliminates or alters normal vaginal bacteria.
- Limit the use of antibiotics during pregnancy and in the postpartum period. If antibiotics are necessary, use a probiotic afterward to replenish your normal bacteria.
- Have a vaginal birth. If you have a cesarean, you can seed the baby with your vaginal bacteria after birth (see page 221).
- Have skin-to-skin contact frequently during the first month of life.
- Breastfeed.
- Bathe the baby with warm plain water only, without any soaps or shampoos.
- Minimize the number of people other than family members who handle the baby during the first few months.

you can place the baby near the breast as well. It will smell and lick the nipple. Suckling usually begins twenty to forty minutes after birth. You do not need to actively insert the nipple into the baby's mouth. In fact, breastfeeding may be more successful if you allow the baby to initiate it. Often, in the hospital setting, a baby will be swaddled and placed next to the mother's breast immediately. However, it is unlikely that a newborn will try to nurse right away. It is better to remove the swaddle, enjoy the skin-to-skin contact, and let the baby find its way to the breast when it is ready.

The Power of the First Impression

In the 1970s, Dr. Frederick Leboyer, a French ob-gyn, first popularized the idea of a baby's gentle transition to the outside world. He advocated placing a newborn in a small bath of warm water, now called the Leboyer bath, to calm the baby. He also believed that to minimize stress, the baby should be massaged and held by its mother in a quiet room with low lights. Leboyer baths are not done regularly anymore, but the philosophy behind them can be carried forward to the modern delivery room.

Whether your labor was fast and furious or slow and exhausting, there is nothing more enjoyable than the first moments with your new baby. The "golden hour" is the time of uninterrupted bonding during the first hour after delivery. Skin-to-skin contact between you and your newborn is ideal. Infants who are allowed to lie naked against their mother's skin cry less, more successfully latch on and nurse, and are better able to regulate their body temperature and blood sugar levels. They are more likely to maintain breastfeeding throughout the first six months. Skin-to-skin contact also allows a baby to be colonized with its mother's bacteria, which help with digestion and immunity. For mothers, direct skin contact with the newborn decreases the incidence of postpartum depression and anxiety. It helps "program" the body and brain for maternal attachment and bonding.

Despite numerous studies proving the benefits of skin-to-skin contact, only 54 percent of babies in the United States experience it. Unfortunately, in some hospitals, the "golden hour" is interrupted by standard procedures that could easily and safely be postponed. Traditionally, as soon as the baby was born, it would be handed off to a nurse or doctor who would examine the baby, take vital signs, give the baby a vitamin K shot, and dress the baby in a diaper and hat. The new mother would lie in the delivery bed, exhausted, trying to get a glimpse of her baby through the bodies hovering around it. Now, with scientific evidence mounting about the importance of the "golden hour," many hospitals are changing their protocols to allow mothers and babies to stay together.

In a birthing center or home birth, your midwife will listen to your baby's heart and lungs and take its vital signs with the baby lying on your chest. She will complete other procedures—such as the vitamin K injection—a few hours later.

Promoting the Golden Hour
- Make sure the room is warm and lights low.
- Dry the baby with a towel and allow it to lie against your bare skin with a blanket covering both of you.
- Make sure you aren't distracted.
- Keep visitors to a minimum.

A Natural Cesarean

Skin-to-skin contact immediately after birth is rare in an operating room. The obstetrician shows the baby to its parents but they are unable to touch him because the doctor is wearing a sterile gown. The infant is handed to the pediatric team and placed in a warmer. The baby's nose and mouth are suctioned. He is dried and stimulated to cry. The baby is weighed on the scale, and then wrapped in a warm blanket. At this point, he is handed to his father to hold as its mother looks on. Normally, a mother will hold her baby for the first time when the surgery is finished—sometimes more than an hour after the birth.

While immediate skin-to-skin contact is challenging during a cesarean, some hospitals are changing their policies to make it a priority. A "natural cesarean" emphasizes the interaction between a new mother and her infant without affecting sterile protocols.

The greatest barriers to skin-to-skin contact are the customs of the operating room itself. A mother is lying on her back with her arms strapped to arm boards. The room itself is cold. The surgical drapes, oxygen tubing, IVs, and monitors hinder the mother's ability to hold her baby safely.

To achieve a natural cesarean, the mother's arms should be left free, the IV poles moved, and the surgical drape adjusted so that the mother's chest is exposed. Warm blankets can be placed over the mother and baby. Sometimes an additional nurse is needed in the OR to help with these procedures. Even though a surgical birth may not be in your original plan, you should consider whether a hospital offers the natural cesarean when you are deciding where to deliver.

Rooming In

The hospital nursery lined with rows of newborns in matching caps became popular in the 1940s so that nurses could get all the babies on the same feeding schedule. Family members would gaze through large glass windows. Even mothers would view their newborn from beyond this barrier. Having the baby in the nursery allowed the mother to enjoy a "mini-vacation" after her hard work.

Since the 1970s, many hospitals offer the option of having your baby "room in," staying with you in your postpartum room. Rooming in is critical to establishing good breastfeeding habits and bonding. Having the baby near you, undisturbed, allows you to notice its subtle nursing cues. However, only 37 percent of newborns are kept with their mothers constantly. The rate of rooming in varies considerably from state to state. In Mississippi and New Jersey, less than 10 percent of babies stay with their mothers while Alaska and Washington have rates near 90 percent.

Of course, your friends and family are excited to meet your new baby. But having lots of visitors during the first few days after delivery can be draining and distracting. You may feel that you need to keep everyone entertained and rehash your birth story over and over. Having one or two family members who can give you a hand is ideal, but ask the others to visit you over the next few weeks when you are home. Don't be afraid to ask people to leave if you are exhausted.

What if you need a break? Should you use the nursery at the hospital? While there is a known benefit to rooming in, some moms need to rest without the stress of taking care of the baby. If you are having significant pain after a cesarean, or if you have been awake for days in labor and feel confused or foggy, a few hours without the baby may make all the difference in your recovery. You can breastfeed, and then move the baby to the nursery so as to clear your mind and get some rest.

The Placenta—Should You Toss It or Eat It?

The placenta is a unique organ that delivers nutrition to your baby and carries away waste. It is composed of lobes, called cotyledons, and weighs just over a pound. Normally, the placenta is discarded after delivery. Recently, placentophagia, eating the placenta, has become a popular trend.

Most mammals, other than humans and marine mammals, eat their placentas. In the wild, eating the placenta is done to eliminate the scent of recent childbirth, so as to protect the young. The placenta can also be a food source for the mother. Dried placenta has been used in Traditional Chinese Medicine (TCM) for hundreds of years to strengthen the body and nourish the blood. The practice has gained popularity recently, as numerous celebrities attest to its benefits.

Ingesting the placenta is believed to help prevent postpartum depression, reduce pain, boost energy, increase lactation, promote skin elasticity, support bonding, and replenish iron stores. Substances commonly found in the placenta during pregnancy, such as estrogen, progesterone, endorphins, iron, and oxytocin, are postulated to have these effects.

While there are many subjective reports and blogs about the benefits of eating the placenta, no medical research supports this practice. Whether the hormones from the placenta are still active after delivery is unknown.

Placental preparation costs $200 to $500. After delivery, you would contact your chosen company, and keep your placenta on ice until it can be picked up. The placenta will be prepared—either raw or encapsulated—and returned to you in the next few days.

the doctor's diary

I have searched long and hard for evidence to support eating the placenta. Honestly, I have. I think it sounds like an interesting thing to do. I have friends who have placental preparation businesses and I want to support them in any way I can. I have looked for any legitimate studies—not just anecdotes of women saying they felt energetic and made lots of breast milk.

Two small studies from the early 1900s mention the practice but draw no conclusions about its benefits. Two other studies were done on pain sensation in rats who ate their placentas. Other than this somewhat marginal research, the only evidence is from the stories of mothers.

I think the subject requires investigation, and a number of questions answered:

- What hormones are actually present in placental tissue postpartum?
- Do hormones "live" in tissue once it is out of the body and there is no blood flowing through it?
- What type of bacteria or enzymes are in the placenta postpartum? Are any of those dangerous?
- If you bake the placenta and put it in capsules, are any of the hormones still active? How would they survive the preparation process?

- Does eating the placenta have a placebo effect? If you expect a therapy to work, it is more likely to do so. If you pay a lot of money for it, the placebo effect is even greater.

A study would be simple enough—give half of the women capsules of placenta and the other half placebo capsules. Measure breast milk production, depression, and the other conditions consuming a placenta is supposed to impact or cure. One website for placental encapsulation says, "Experts agree that the placenta retains hormones, and thus reintroducing them to your system may ease hormonal fluctuations." Yet I cannot find any research to back up these statements and I'm not sure who these "experts" are.

While the benefits of eating the placenta haven't been proven, the risks appear to be minimal. We have not yet seen any outbreak of infections from this practice. If it isn't dangerous, and you believe it will help, then it may be worth a try. Midwives and doulas attest to their personal experience of new moms feeling better and coping with the postpartum transition with ease after ingesting the placenta.

The jury is still out on this one!

The Postpartum Baby

Regardless of how your baby was born, some routine procedures are done to make sure the baby is healthy. While these tests and treatments are recommended, ultimately, it is your decision whether they are performed. Since some of these are done immediately after delivery, make sure your doctor and the hospital staff know your wishes.

Routine Suctioning

Suctioning the baby with a bulb syringe during the first few minutes of life removes mucus and amniotic fluid from its nose and mouth. However, suctioning an infant who is vigorously crying is unnecessary because the cry itself has the same effect. It may even be harmful because it triggers a reflex that lowers the baby's heart rate and suppresses breathing.

Many physicians perform this procedure out of habit, while midwives are less likely to suction babies routinely. If you are delivering with an OB, you can request that your baby is only suctioned if medically necessary.

Vitamin K Injection

Vitamin K plays a critical role in blood clotting. Half of all infants are vitamin K deficient in the first six months of life. Attempting to boost your own vitamin K stores during pregnancy has little effect on your baby's vitamin K levels because it doesn't easily cross the placenta. One percent of babies with low vitamin K will have bleeding from the umbilical cord site, the nose, the intestines, or within the brain. Unfortunately, there are no warning signs that a life-threatening event is about to take place. Since 1961, an injection of vitamin K has been given routinely to newborns within six hours of birth, essentially eliminating the risk of bleeding.

In the United States, vitamin K is only available as an injection. In other countries, while the injection is preferred, it can also be given orally as a liquid in multiple doses over three months. This has not been an option in the United States because the oral form is not as effective and doctors fear that patients won't receive all three doses. The injection may be uncomfortable for your newborn, but there are no other consequences.

Numerous studies attest to the safety of this vitamin. Nonetheless, many websites falsely claim that it causes cancer or question its necessity. Others say that your baby will have "psycho-emotional damage and trauma" from the injection itself, though there is no reliable evidence to support this notion. Nearly all babies born in a hospital receive the vitamin K injection. However only 70 percent of babies born in birthing centers or at home receive it.

After delivery, if you decline the vitamin K injection and plan to breastfeed exclusively, you can take a vitamin K supplement (2.5 mg twice per day) to increase the levels in your breast milk. In addition, some women use the liquid from the injection as an oral treatment for the baby. The regimen is 2 to 4 mg at birth followed by 2 mg at four and eight weeks of life. Oral vitamin K supplements are available for purchase on the Internet but are not regulated by the FDA, so there is no way to guarantee how much of the vitamin the baby would actually receive. Infant formula contains an ample amount of vitamin K so there are virtually no cases of bleeding in formula-fed babies.

Erythromycin Eye Drops

The American Academy of Pediatrics recommends applying erythromycin ointment to the eyes of all babies after delivery to prevent eye infections that can cause blindness, whether the baby was born vaginally or by cesarean. The antibiotic ointment is a gooey gel applied to the eyelids. Other than mild swelling around the eye, there are no major side effects to the treatment.

Medications have been used in the United States for over one hundred years to prevent these infections, which are caused by gonorrhea and chlamydia. Currently, thirty-two states have laws dating back to the early 1900s that mandate this procedure.

While erythromycin is a safe and simple therapy, there may be some circumstances in which you can reasonably decline it. For example, if you had a cesarean and your water bag was never broken, the baby isn't exposed to any vaginal bacteria. In addition, if you have tested negative for chlamydia and gonorrhea during pregnancy, and are in a monogamous relationship, your baby isn't at risk. Another option, practiced in the United Kingdom, is to administer the antibiotic if the baby shows signs of an eye infection.

Check with your provider about your hospital or birthing center's policies. Many will allow you to sign a refusal for the procedure.

Hepatitis B Vaccine

Since 2002, the American Academy of Pediatrics recommends that all newborns receive the hepatitis B vaccine before discharge from the hospital. This is the only vaccine that is offered in the immediate postpartum period.

Hepatitis B is a liver infection that can cause cirrhosis and liver cancer. Whereas many adults who are exposed to hepatitis B will clear the infection, infants and young children are more likely to carry the disease throughout their lives. The infection is passed sexually, through contaminated needles, or from an infected mother to her baby during childbirth. Sharing a toothbrush can also spread hepatitis. The virus can live on a surface for seven days, so a child crawling on the floor of a daycare where an infected child has been playing can become infected by putting hands or toys in its mouth.

This vaccine is given immediately after birth so as to protect the newborn from exposure to hepatitis B from well-meaning family and friends who love to kiss and snuggle with the baby. In addition, pediatricians believe that, if the family starts the vaccination series at birth, they are more likely to complete the full course, two additional shots that are given at two months and six months.

Many new parents assume they don't know anyone with hepatitis B, so being vaccinated isn't important for their baby. However, 1.2 million Americans have this infection. The vaccine has been given to newborns since 1991 with no adverse effects. Hepatitis B vaccination after delivery may be waived by signing a refusal in the medical record. You should speak with your pediatrician before delivery about your wishes.

The First Bath

In the past, a baby received its first bath in the delivery room or in the nursery shortly after birth. Nurses would wash the baby, swaddle it, and hand it to its mother in a perfect, clean package. As the benefits of colonizing the baby's microbiome have been discovered, mothers are choosing to postpone this procedure.

Vernix, the white, creamy substance that coats the skin, serves to waterproof the baby, preventing its skin from wrinkling during pregnancy. It also helps the newborn stay warm and fight off unwanted infections, such as Group B strep and *E. coli*. Vernix can be massaged into the skin like a lotion.

The World Health Organization (WHO) now recommends delaying bathing until twenty-four hours after delivery. By waiting, the baby has a reduced risk of infection, stabilized blood sugar levels, and improved temperature control. It also improves breast-feeding rates because it allows uninterrupted time for mother and baby together. The baby should be washed with warm, plain water. No soap or shampoo is needed. Watching a nurse give the baby a first bath in the hospital before discharge can be helpful for new parents to learn the technique, but it is also perfectly fine to wait until you are home.

Circumcision

Circumcision, a surgical procedure that removes the foreskin from the penis, began in ancient Egypt either as a religious tradition, or to mark the transition from boyhood to manhood. For thousands of years, it continued as an initiation ritual or as a religious obligation. More recently, circumcision was performed for reasons of health and hygiene, though its benefits are disputed.

Today, the United States is the only developed country where infant boys are routinely circumcised for nonreligious reasons. About 70 percent of infants undergo this procedure, usually the day after birth. The rates of circumcision vary widely: In the Midwest it is 75 percent, whereas on the West Coast it is only 30 percent. Caucasians are circumcised a higher rate (91 percent) than are African

Americans (73 percent) or Hispanics (44 percent). In the United Kingdom, the rate is 16 percent; Canada, 50 percent; and Australia, 9 percent.

The most common reasons that a family chooses to circumcise:

- Concerns about hygiene
- Family tradition
- Religious reasons

The Controversy over the Procedure

Many medical organizations, including the WHO, advocate circumcision because the procedure is good for public health, especially with its benefits of decreasing the spread of such STDs as human immunodeficiency virus (HIV) and human papillomavirus (HPV). The results of several studies—the validity of which are disputed by anticircumcision groups—show that circumcision reduced the rate of heterosexual transmission of HIV by 60 percent. The American Academy of Pediatrics says that the health benefits outweigh its risks, but that a family can ultimately make its own choice. However, others say that it is unethical to make this kind of a decision for a baby, when the medical benefits are minor. Circumcised men have described permanent emotional scarring from having a procedure that they did not consent to.

Benefits of Circumcision

- Fewer urinary tract infections (UTIs): Circumcision reduces the incidence of UTIs by 90 percent. However, these infections are quite rare, only happening in 1 in 100 infants. Over a lifetime, an uncircumcised man is 4 times more likely to get a UTI than a circumcised man is.
- Less penile cancer: Penile cancer occurs in 1 in 100,000 men, but occurs less in circumcised men.
- Less cervical cancer in female partners: Cervical cancer is more common in women who have uncircumcised part-

ners. HPV, which causes abnormal Pap smears and cervical cancer, lives in the foreskin. Men who are uncircumcised are 3 times more likely to carry HPV.

- Reduction in HIV and herpes: Circumcision decreases the spread of HIV and herpes. However, it does not affect the transmission of chlamydia, gonorrhea, or syphilis.
- Easier hygiene: Uncircumcised men must wash beneath the foreskin to maintain good hygiene.

Disadvantages of Circumcision

- Complications: Complications of the procedure itself occur in 0.2 percent of babies. These include bleeding, infection, injury to the penis, and scarring.
- Pain from the procedure: Infants are less interactive and eat less for the first 24 hours after circumcision. However, this is not seen if topical anesthesia is used.
- Sexual dissatisfaction: The foreskin covers the end of the penis. It is possible that when the glans is uncovered, it will become less sensitive, and sex will be less pleasurable.

Hearing Test

One to 2 babies in 1,000 are born with permanent hearing loss, usually as a result of a genetic mutation. A baby can be screened for hearing loss on the day after birth. A sound—usually a click or tone—is played near the baby's ear though an earphone. Through an electrode placed on the baby's forehead, a doctor can determine whether the baby heard the sound.

Testing for Jaundice

Jaundice is a condition in which bilirubin, a breakdown product of red blood cells, builds up in the blood and makes the skin appear yellow. Mild jaundice occurs in 84 percent of normal newborns, and is the most common reason that a baby is readmitted to a hospital after birth. Two percent of newborns will develop severe jaundice, which can cause brain damage. The American Academy of Pediatrics recommends that all babies be screened for jaundice before they are discharged from the hospital. Screening may be done with a blood sample or with a handheld device that measures the bilirubin level in the skin.

In the first week after birth, check your baby's face, eyes, and soles of the feet for yellow discoloration by laying your child on a white sheet. Contact your pediatrician if you are concerned.

Babies who are at higher risk for jaundice are those who were born before thirty-seven weeks, have a sibling with history of jaundice, have a different blood type than their mother, or were born with the assistance of a vacuum or forceps.

Preventing Jaundice

When a baby drinks fluids, the bilirubin is flushed out of its blood. You should breastfeed eight to twelve times per day during the first few days of life. If an infant is severely dehydrated, sugar water may be used in addition to breast milk. Putting your baby in the sunlight for a few minutes every day does not prevent jaundice; it would take hours of this exposure to make a significant change in bilirubin levels, and would not be safe.

If Your Baby Has Jaundice

Feeding your baby frequently is the best way to treat mild jaundice. Breastfeeding can almost always be continued as long as the bilirubin levels don't continue to rise.

Phototherapy—the use of a special fluorescent light to break down the bilirubin in the skin—is a treatment for babies with high bilirubin. The therapy, prescribed by a doctor, can be done in a hospital or at home with portable lights or a fiber-optic blanket called a bili-blanket. Treatment usually lasts for twenty-four hours or longer. During therapy, the baby should be uncovered under the lights as much as possible, and removed only temporarily to feed and be changed. Your doctor will check the bilirubin level every day and stop the light treatment when the level has declined.

Newborn Blood Screening

All states require screening of newborns for a variety of serious medical conditions, such as phenylketonuria and congenital hypo-thyroidism, that have no symptoms at birth. The specific tests in the screening panel vary from state to state. If your baby tests positive, treatments need to be undertaken immediately.

The screening should be done when the baby is twenty-four to forty-eight hours old. A few drops of blood are collected via a heel stick. The results will be sent to your pediatrician in two weeks. Although opting out of this screening is highly discouraged, parents can do so for religious reasons by signing a waiver.

Feeding Your Baby

Breastfeeding is the most economical feeding method, offering the most nutrients in an easily digestible form for your new baby. While it should come naturally, for thousands of years, women have struggled with nursing and have sought ways to produce more milk. *The Papyrus Ebers*, the earliest medical encyclope-dia from Egypt in 1550 BC, describes a method to help a woman breastfeed. It says: "To get a supply of milk in a woman's breast for suckling a child: Warm the bones of a swordfish in oil and rub her back with it."[1]

Benefits of Breastfeeding

Breast milk is the optimal food source for the first year of life be-cause it contains nutrients, as well as enzymes, growth factors, and antibodies that science hasn't been able to replicate in formula.

Breastfeeding reduces the risk of ear infections, dermatitis, respiratory infections, childhood leukemia, asthma, sudden infant death syndrome (SIDS), and diabetes.

Newborns are susceptible to infections because their immune system is immature. Some antibodies are passed to the fetus through the placenta during the last three months of pregnancy, but these antibodies wane in the first few weeks of life. Breast milk contains additional antibodies to fight disease until the baby's immune system can produce its own, when the baby is two months old. Therefore, breastfeeding even for only eight weeks can give a tremendous advantage to your baby.

Establishing Breastfeeding

Preparation for breastfeeding begins at the onset of pregnancy. The breast glands enlarge and colostrum, the premilk, is made after sixteen weeks. After delivery of the baby and placenta, estrogen and progesterone levels fall and prolactin rises, triggering breast milk production. These hormonal changes takes place over seventy-two hours. As a result, you will have a full milk supply after three days, no matter the route of delivery or frequency of nursing. Colostrum is available during this time. Although the volume produced is small—just over an ounce per day—it is full of antibodies that protect your baby from infections.

The most important factors in sustaining milk production are the frequency and duration of nursing. Nursing should be done every two to three hours. If your baby is asleep, you should empty the breast with a pump. The breast must be completely emptied at each feeding. If milk remains in the breast, your body thinks that the baby is satisfied and less milk will be produced.

Aspects of your labor and the early postpartum period influence your ability to breastfeed. A baby has reflexes that signal that it is ready to nurse almost immediately after birth, such as moving its hands toward its mouth and sucking on its fists. If a baby was exposed to high levels of Pitocin during labor, fewer of these prefeeding behaviors are seen. The use of opiate pain medications, such as Demerol and Stadol, make it harder for the baby to coordinate the sucking motions needed to draw milk from the breast. Having your baby room in allows you to learn your newborn's breastfeeding cues. Ideally you should feed your baby when it first shows the feeding behaviors, such as opening its mouth. If it isn't fed promptly, the baby will become fussy, kicking its feet, and eventually crying loudly. Once the baby is agitated, latching on properly is more difficult. Overstimulation of the baby with exams, eye treatments, and injections may cause some babies to become jittery, unable to focus, and distracted from the instinctive behaviors. Therefore, you should minimize activities that don't need to be done immediately, to allow your baby to transition to the outside world, and to breastfeeding, peacefully.

Nipple Confusion

Nipple confusion occurs when a baby tries to nurse from the breast with the same technique used to nurse from an artificial nipple. At the breast, a contraction wave moves from the tip of the tongue to the back, massaging the milk out of the nipple. With a bottle, the baby's mouth squeezes the milk out like a piston. If a baby becomes accustomed to a bottle, it may have difficulty sucking from the breast. Nipple confusion most commonly occurs if an artificial nipple from a bottle or pacifier is offered before breastfeeding is well established, usually within the first three weeks.

Some mothers choose to give their baby breast milk out of a bottle instead of nursing. This way, the mother can pump milk every two to four hours and prepare bottles of milk for when she is out or at work. Having pumped milk also gives partners and other family members a way to be involved in feeding the baby.

Women Who Can't Nurse

Although breastfeeding has benefits, women with certain medical conditions cannot breastfeed.

- HIV: Because HIV is passed through breast milk, women who are HIV positive should not breastfeed.
- Breast-reduction surgery: After breast-reduction surgery in which the nipple has been removed and repositioned, it is nearly impossible to nurse because the nipple is no longer attached to the breast glands underneath.
- Hypoplastic breast glands: Some women—those with tubular-shaped breasts—don't have enough breast glands to produce milk.
- Medications: Women taking such medications as chemotherapy or radioactive iodine cannot breastfeed.
- Metabolic disorders in the newborn: Babies with PKU and galactosemia may not be able to nurse. These diseases are detected through the newborn screening tests. If your baby has one of these disorders, talk to your pediatrician to see whether nursing is safe.

How to Know Whether You Are Making Enough Milk

During the first month, you should nurse eight to twelve times per day. Nursing should begin when the baby shows the early breastfeeding cues, or if more than four hours has passed.

Signs that you have a good milk supply:

- Your baby is calm and satisfied.
- When the baby is full, it will naturally detach from the nipple.

- Your baby is gaining weight. A baby will normally lose 5 to 7 percent of its birth weight during the first few days, but should be back to its original weight within one to two weeks.

Why Women Stop Nursing

According to Centers for Disease Control (CDC) data from 2011, 77 percent of US newborns begin breastfeeding, 49 percent are still nursing at six months, and 27 percent at twelve months. Commitment to exclusive breastfeeding for six months as suggested by the American Academy of Pediatrics is particularly challenging in a country without paid maternity leave and policies to help new families. These days, breastfeeding is more common for women who are wealthy and lowest for women below the poverty line. Poor women have the least support and may work in jobs where they are unable to pump milk for the baby to drink in their absence. They may also need to return to work sooner after delivery.

Most women who use midwives breastfeed, although the exact reason why is unclear. It could be that women who choose a midwife are already planning on nursing. A midwife may give extra assistance that a doctor wouldn't, and the birth environment with a midwife—with less intervention—makes it easier to initiate nursing.

Inadequate breast milk production, caused by stress, anxiety, or fatigue, is a common reason women stop nursing. Stress inhibits the release of oxytocin, so less milk is produced. A mother will resort to supplementing with formula, followed by less nursing, and even less production.

While some women say, "My milk never came in," nearly every mother can nurse given the proper support, training, and time. Poor feeding routines, such as nursing in uncomfortable positions or attempting to nurse for only a few minutes, also lead to reduced milk production. If the baby doesn't latch on well or falls asleep during nursing, new moms can become frustrated and give up.

Techniques for Promoting Breastfeeding

- Ask to see a lactation consultant while you are in the hospital and/or hire one for when you are home.
- Don't be tempted by the "gift" of formula in your room.
- Find a relaxing, comfortable position for nursing.
- Stay well hydrated.
- Eliminate distractions during nursing. Turn off the TV and play some soft music instead.
- Nurse alone, or only with your partner present, so that you don't feel self-conscious or anxious about being observed.
- Empty each breast completely.
- After the breast has been emptied by the baby, attach a pump for an extra 10 minutes. Although little milk will be expressed, it will trick your body into thinking the baby is still feeding. Over the next week, you will produce more milk.
- Limit the use of pacifiers and bottles, especially in the first 3 weeks.

Supplements and Medications for Increasing Milk Production

Agents to increase milk production, called galactagogues, range from herbal supplements to prescription drugs and even to beer. Galactagogues should only be used after traditional methods for increasing milk supply have not been effective. Scientific evidence supporting the use of any galactagogues—herbal and prescription—is sparse at best.

Beer: Women have tried to increase breast milk supply by drinking beer for a few hundred years. In the early 1900s, Anheuser-Busch even produced beer specifically for nursing mothers, called Malt Nutrine. However, medical studies don't show an overall benefit to drinking beer. While the hops and barley in beer increase prolactin production, the alcohol decreases it. Overall, infants consume 20 percent less milk in the three to four hours after a mother's alcohol consumption. The hops from nonalcoholic beers have the same effect on prolactin without the disadvantage of the alcohol.

Domperidone: Domperidone is a prescription medication used to treat nausea that raises prolactin levels, doubling milk production. The dosage of domperidone is 10 mg three times per day. It does not affect the baby. For the mother, side effects include a dry mouth, headache, or itching.

Despite its proven benefits, domperidone is not available in the United States because of a concern about a rare side effect, an irregular heartbeat, seen in women with heart disease when the drug is taken in high doses. In 2004, the FDA made ordering domperidone from pharmacies in other countries illegal and instructed US customs agents to confiscate it. In addition, compounding pharmacies can be fined for producing it. Domperidone is used regularly in other parts of the world. In some countries, such as the United Kingdom and Japan, it is even available without a prescription.

Fenugreek: Fenugreek is an herb used to flavor maple syrup and curry powder. By stimulating sweat glands to produce more fluid, anecdotal evidence suggests that it increases milk production within a few days. Fenugreek is supplied in 500 mg capsules. The typical dosage is three capsules three times per day, 4,500 mg per day total. Women using fenugreek notice that their urine, milk, and perspiration smell like maple syrup.

Milk thistle: Milk thistle, with its active ingredient silymarin, is a plant that has been used to increase milk production for generations. The recommended dosage is 420 mg of silymarin per day.

Oxytocin: The hormone oxytocin causes the muscles around the milk glands to squeeze the milk out, thoroughly emptying the breast so the glands are stimulated to produce more milk. While studies are limited, one shows milk volume is two to five times higher for mothers using oxytocin.

Oxytocin is no longer available from regular pharmacies because the FDA says there isn't enough evidence about its effectiveness. With a prescription from your doctor, some compounding pharmacies supply oxytocin as a nasal spray (40 U/ml). You use one spray per nostril prior to nursing. There are no known side effects for mother or baby. Over-the-counter products claiming to contain "oxytocin" should not be trusted. True oxytocin is only available by prescription.

Reglan: Reglan is an antinausea medication that increases prolactin production and breast milk volume. The dosage is 10 mg orally three times per day. Side effects include headaches, depression, and fatigue in the mother and mild stomach upset in the newborn. Data from research studies are mixed about its effectiveness.

Eating and Drinking When You Are Nursing

Human milk is composed of lactose (milk sugar), fat, protein, vitamins, and minerals. While you are nursing, you should eat a well-balanced diet. There are no specific foods that you need to avoid. Production of breast milk requires 500 calories per day. About 200 calories are obtained from your fat stores, so you need to consume an extra 300 calories while nursing.

Some medications may decrease milk production, including antihistamines, decongestants, hormonal contraceptives with estrogen, and nicotine. To be safe, check with your doctor before using over-the-counter medications while you are breastfeeding.

A pet peeve of mine: the websites and pregnancy books that list end-less foods that you can't eat while nursing. Chocolate, citrus, peanuts, eggs, parsley—the lists go on and on, with no medical evidence what-soever! No matter what, your baby will have days of fussiness and days of calm. You may try to attribute the fussy days to something you ate, but it is actually just the normal fluctuations of your baby's maturing digestive system.

Foods that cause gas in a mother, such as broccoli or beans, do not cause gas in a baby. Gas is caused by the interaction of intestinal bacteria and fiber in certain foods. Breast milk does not contain fiber or gas. Instead, gassiness in a baby is due to its immature digestive system, consuming milk too fast, or crying while trying to eat.

What you eat while nursing does not cause allergies in your baby. There is no reason to avoid certain foods, such as nuts, dairy, or eggs, be-cause you think your baby will become allergic to them. In fact, breast-feeding has been shown to reduce the risk of food allergies through the teenage years.

Drinking alcohol and coffee in moderation while nursing is safe. Alco-hol levels in the blood and breast milk peak thirty to forty-five minutes after drinking and the amount that actually passes to the baby is in-significant. It can, however, slightly alter some babies' sleep patterns, such that they sleep more frequently but for shorter intervals. Caffeine, from coffee, tea, or chocolate, does not affect your baby unless the amount is significant. Up to three cups of coffee per day is safe for breastfeeding mothers.

Where to Find Lactation Advice

Seventy percent of new mothers admit that they receive breastfeed-ing advice from the media or on the Internet, but studies show at least 25 percent of this advice is wrong. Should you have trouble with breastfeeding, there are specialists who can help you. Ask your doctor, nurse, or midwife for a recommendation for a lactation consultant.

My postpartum patients in the hospital tell me that they hear conflicting advice about nursing. Their nurse during the day says one thing, the night nurse another, the doula has another opinion, and the doctor still one more. Very little instruction is given during an ob-gyn's residency to prepare us to be experts on breastfeeding. Personally, I was not taught anything about helping women to nurse or how to increase milk production. The only information I received was from observing some of the experienced postpartum nurses.

About 20 percent of mothers say their doctors gave them no advice at all; and when they did, the messages were sometimes contradictory to those they got from nurses and lactation specialists. Some doctors and nurses are quick to suggest supplementing with formula at the slightest hint of a problem, saying, "There is no reason to torture yourself." Lactation consultants, on the other hand, may tell worried mothers to "try harder." Neither suggestion helps a new mom feel much better.

Lactation consultants are certified through the International Board of Lactation Consultant Examiners (IBLCE). They complete a 90-hour course, obtain 500 to 1,000 hours of clinical experience, and pass an exam. You can find a consultant in your area at www.ilca. org. Since the adoption of the Affordable Care Act, health insurance plans (though not all states' Medicaid plans) must cover the cost of lactation consultants as well as breast pumps without copayment. You can contact your insurance plan directly to find information about which pumps are covered and which lactation consultants are part of your network. You may also be able to receive a free pump through the Women, Infants, and Children (WIC) program.

The Popularity of Formula

Synthetic formula was invented over one hundred years ago as an alternative for babies whose mothers had died in childbirth. From the 1940s through the 1970s, only 25 percent of women in the United States nursed. At that time, formula was touted as convenient, especially for women who had entered the workforce. At that time, women who breastfed were predominantly low-income. Despite the popularity of formula, scientific evidence persuaded the American Academy of Pediatrics to recommend breastfeeding over formula for the first time in 1978.

Baby formula is a $5 billion per year industry. Formula manufacturers market directly to consumers via gift bags of formula and coupons that are given to women after delivery in the hospital. As a result, many new moms believe that the hospital is endorsing formula and they are less likely to breastfeed. A recent campaign, Ban the Bags, is attempting to eliminate these gifts. From 2007 to 2013, the percentage of hospitals giving gift bags of formula has decreased from 73 to 32 percent. Nonetheless, 24 percent of breastfed infants received formula during their hospital stay.

The WIC program, which began in the 1970s, provides low-income women and children with nutritious food. While it sponsors numerous programs on the benefits of breastfeeding, it also provides formula for half of the infants born in the United States every year.

the doctor's diary

Of course, mothers want to do everything they can to support their children. But what if, for whatever reason, you have chosen to formula-feed? I'm here to assure you that all is not lost.

Most studies on the long-term benefits of breast milk versus formula compare children in different families and different parts of the country. A 2014 study instead looked at the long-term health and well-being of siblings—genetically related and living under the same roof—where some were breastfed and the others formula-fed.[2] The data show that there was no difference in long-term well-being, including obesity, reading, memory, and parental bonding. Instead, the authors concluded that some of the benefits that have been attributed to breast milk may actually be due to a family's overall healthy habits.

While breastfeeding is associated with higher IQs, it is not an ingredient in the milk that makes children smarter. Instead, a breastfeeding mom responds to her baby's emotional cues better and is more likely to read to her baby earlier in life.[3] She may be at home for a longer time before she returns to work. So, it's not the milk—it's the parenting.

The more proper hygiene and nutrition, the more talking and reading to children, and the more exercising, the less breastfeeding seems to matter. Good parenting can overcome some of the potential 'deficits' for a formula-fed child.

The debate over breastfeeding versus formula has strong defenders on each side. Breastfeeding is portrayed as the ultimate expression of maternal dedication. Women who don't do it are seen as bad mothers and called selfish. Some new moms miss out on the joy of motherhood because they are stressed and guilt-ridden about breastfeeding. Instead of prolonging the debate over breast milk versus formula, we should focus our energy on training counselors to help families with whatever they decide. Promoting parental behaviors that improve child development, such as reading to children, holding them, and talking to them, will help them thrive, no matter how they are fed. Isn't it better to support new moms in any way possible?

Breastfeeding, Formula Feeding, or a Little of Both

For many mothers, especially those who need to go back to work shortly after delivery, breast milk and formula may be the perfect combination. Any amount of breast milk is beneficial. But if you find that your supply declines due to a work schedule or a baby who doesn't latch well, using a bottle of formula to satisfy a hungry infant is absolutely acceptable.

Postpartum Depression

Nearly everyone feels emotional after delivery. A roller coaster of joy and elation can be followed by sadness and anxiety. The line between a normal emotional wave and depression can be difficult to draw.

One quarter of women have emotional changes that can be classified as postpartum depression (PPD), although less than 15 percent of these women seek treatment. PPD includes feelings of despair and hopelessness, exhaustion, anxiety over small details, and guilt that, although the baby is healthy, you still aren't happy. If you have suicidal thoughts or ideas of hurting your baby, you need to see a medical professional immediately.

The sudden drop in estrogen and progesterone at delivery is linked to PPD. This change in hormone levels combined with sleep deprivation, stress, lack of support, or a demanding baby turn normal sadness into depression. The "baby blues" are feelings of anxiety and restlessness that occur within the first two weeks of delivery, and then resolve. Postpartum depression may grow out of the baby blues, or start anytime within the first year after delivery.

Women with a history of depression and anxiety are at increased risk of PPD, but it can happen to anyone. It is also more common in women who have had postpartum depression with a previous pregnancy, those with a weak support system, an unplanned pregnancy, or a history of physical abuse before or during pregnancy. Women with the most prenatal care visits, those who took sick leave during pregnancy, and those who have had difficulty breastfeeding also suffer from depression more often.

Studies of other cultures show that postpartum depression is rare in non-Western societies. Scientists believe that the lack of postpartum rituals and minimal family or community involvement in the birth experience contribute to depression. In Western societies, there is more physical fatigue, uncertainty about social support, and stress on the relationship with a partner. Cultures with structured postpartum practices and rituals ease the mother into her maternal role.

Screening for PPD

New guidelines in 2015 urge physicians and midwives to screen all of their postpartum patients for depression. The Edinburgh Postpartum Depression Scale–3 is a simple questionnaire that may indicate when further investigation is necessary.[4] A score of 6 or more is associated with PPD. Here is the scale so you can screen yourself.

Ask yourself how you have been feeling in the last seven days:

1. I have blamed myself unnecessarily when things have gone wrong.
   3 Most of the time
   2 Some of the time
   1 Not very often
   0 Never
2. I have been anxious or nervous for no good reason.
   3 Very often
   2 Sometimes
   1 Hardly ever
   0 Not at all
3. I felt scared or panicky for no good reason.
   3 Quite a lot
   2 Sometimes
   1 Not much
   0 Not at all

Treatment for PPD

New moms and their partners should be aware of the signs of depression and seek help from their general doctor or obstetrician. Treatment for postpartum depression includes therapy, medications, or both. Many antidepressants can be taken safely while breastfeeding.

Dealing With a Birth That Didn't Go as Planned

Meeting all the goals of your birth plan is one way to feel satisfied with your delivery. But even women who end up with an unexpected cesarean can walk away fulfilled. How you feel also depends on how you were treated during the decision-making process. Birth trauma stems from situations that veered out of control, such that the mother didn't feel as if she had any say in what was happening. She carries the weight of that experience with her through the postpartum period.

the doctor's diary

One third of women describes their birth as traumatic. Every birth has its ups and downs, but I am always disheartened to hear how many women have a birth story that is negative. While the majority of these experiences still led to a healthy baby, the mother is nonetheless affected. If you believe your birth was mismanaged, you may be angry. You may also feel embarrassed that you didn't stick to a birth plan, asked for an epidural, or had a cesarean because the baby wouldn't come out.

When I walk into a room to make my postpartum rounds at the hospital, I am never sure what to expect. Some moms are simply giddy with excitement, but others tell me they are disappointed about what happened the day before. They want to go over the details with me, or ask questions about how things could have been done differently. The feelings about their birth set the tone for the first few days and weeks with their new baby. I hope that our discussion can give them a sense of peace and confidence to move forward.

Causes of Birth Trauma

- Unexpected cesarean
- Heavy bleeding after delivery
- Pain from an episiotomy or laceration
- Baby's going to the neonatal intensive care unit (NICU)
- Poor communication
- Unhelpful or dismissive hospital staff
- Having a procedure without adequate consent
- Cesarean or vaginal birth without adequate pain relief (an ineffective epidural)
- Being yelled at for "pushing wrong"
- Feeling like a failure for not being able to push the baby out
- Feeling that your priorities were dismissed

Dealing with a Negative Experience

Thankfully, most women and their babies are physically healthy after delivery. In our culture, we expect mothers to be grateful and joyful when their baby is born. Friends and family may not understand why a mother feels frustrated or disappointed.

But birth stays with us. It is not just another day. You will remember what the weather was like and what you were doing when labor started. The narrative of your birth will be repeated to friends and family, and will be replayed in your mind many times over. The story defines who you are as a mother and the details influence your ability to parent. If you have a positive experience, you leave the hospital feeling confident and strong. If you had a bad experience, you may have uncertainty and doubt about your ability to take care of your baby.

How to Cope

- Talk about the experience with friends.
- Try hypnosis.
- See a therapist.
- Allow yourself time to grieve.
- Trust that you are a good mother. The way you gave birth has nothing to do with your ability to be your baby's best caretaker.
- Write about the experience.
- Talk to your provider about what happened. It is okay to let him know you are angry or disappointed. Your provider needs to review the details with you, acknowledging that your experience was traumatic and that your pain is real.

Remember that sometimes a birth that didn't go as planned serves to teach an important lesson—that mothering requires being flexible and yielding to powers beyond us.

⊰ JILL'S STORY ⊱

I just wanted the pregnancy to be healthy and as free of stress as possible since I was also helping to take care of my mom who had terminal cancer. I wanted the labor to result in a healthy baby and mom first and foremost, but I also hoped that I would be able to avoid a C-section. No one wants to be recovering from surgery during the time she is bonding with her new baby and I wanted to know what it felt like to have a vaginal birth. To this end, I also wanted to minimize the use of interventions, like Pitocin, that I thought could complicate the road to a healthy natural birth and increase discomfort during labor. In terms of pain control, I was open to anything. I had heard stories of epidurals making vaginal birth harder but others that made it possible.

I wanted some say in how things were going to happen. I wanted to understand what was going on. I had some distant hope that maybe I would enjoy it or, at least, it wouldn't be that bad. There is so much talk about labor pain; you just wish it won't be as bad as everyone says.

Although I didn't really know what to expect, I did as much preparation as I could. I took my prenatal vitamins, tried to stay active and positive, talked to my family about my goals, toured the hospital, took a birthing class, and hired a doula.

Things did not go as expected. I had a rapid labor and was fully dilated in only a few hours—this was very different from everything I'd read and didn't match with all the preparation I had done. I was planning to see how things went in terms of using pain control. However, once in labor, I was confused about what was the best thing to do. I was in a lot of pain given the labor was progressing so quickly so I took the epidural. I almost felt sad when the pain went away completely; I suddenly detached from the experience. And I hated the feeling of having my legs numb and not being able to move around, but they were able to turn down the epidural and made that a little better.

Of course, there were some benefits from the pain control, too. It was really nice to have some downtime to rest for everyone involved. I remember peaceful moments that were only possible because of the epidural, when I was able to say hi to my mom and dad.

Because I dilated so quickly, my baby's head got stuck in an unusual position. Despite my best efforts, it could not be dislodged, and I needed a cesarean. In the operating room, things really took a turn for the worse. I could feel what the doctors were doing, so the anesthesiologist gave me ketamine. I wish he had been more patient by letting the epidural take effect instead of giving me the ketamine, or at least I wish he had communicated with me what the drug does so I would have understood why I was feeling so weird. After all the communication in the labor room, once I got to the operating room, it ended. The ketamine was the worst part of the whole thing because I was so drugged by the time my baby was actually born that I wasn't able to experience it. Also, I couldn't hear properly because my ears were buzzing, so I couldn't confirm that everything was okay with him once he was born. I heard his cry like it was a million miles away.

Then, because I didn't understand what was happening to me, I seemed nervous, so the anesthesiologist gave me a dose of another medication that was supposed to help me relax but instead caused me to be sick to my stomach for a long time. I suppose I should have made a point of talking to the anesthesiologist ahead of time, after the epidural or before the C-section.

I was thrilled with being a mom and very happy overall, but when I thought about the birth, I was sad that I had a C-section and I was sad that it felt so traumatic. It was all over very quickly and settled back to a feeling of "Okay, everything is going fine." But his birth will always be a weird memory, rather than a sweet memory.

In the end, I was sad that the communication wasn't better. I was sad that something got in the way of me being able to fully experience the birth of my son. I was sad that I was among those that ended up needing a C-section. I had some lingering thought of, "Was there something else we could have done to avoid this?"

I was hoping I would get a chance to fix the things that went wrong with the first birth with my second child, and maybe even be able to have a vaginal delivery. That is always the hope—a quick vaginal birth with no complications.

What is more interesting however, is how my second pregnancy and birth affected my feelings about my first. My second baby was born two and a half months early due to unexpected preterm labor. I had to have another cesarean because my baby was breech and quite small. The C-section was the least traumatic aspect of that birth. Spending two months in the NICU, fearing for my second son's life, reading about his chances for mental impairment and a host of other potential problems, made the cesarean pale in comparison. I was faced with not knowing for a very long time whether he was going to be okay and then also had the difficult task of caring for a preemie along with a toddler who still needed my attention.

These days, I look back on my first son's birth as wonderful. The disappointment about having a C-section and the other things that didn't go as I planned seems trivial. Meeting other parents in the NICU who had even more dire circumstances with their babies than I did with mine and ultimately watching my second son thrive made me feel so lucky and grateful.

After becoming a parent, you share stories with your friends and other moms. You hear about their difficulties getting pregnant, problems during pregnancy, and emergency deliveries. You learn that lots of moms struggle with breastfeeding, have children who were born with mental disabilities or serious diseases. . . . It just seems that, with all that is out there to worry about, if everyone eventually goes home healthy, regardless of the bumps along the way, it is a reason to celebrate. 🖘

Your Body After Having a Baby

According to researchers from the University of Michigan, the single most traumatic event your body will go through during your lifetime is childbirth, which is even more physically stressful than running a marathon. The many physical changes during your pregnancy and delivery can have lasting effects. While you are tending to your newborn, you will also need to care for yourself.

Perineal Care

After delivery, your perineum will be painful and swollen, even if you didn't have an episiotomy or tear. The pain is the greatest for the first few days but can last for a few weeks. Ice packs and ibuprofen decrease the swelling. Arnica, calendula, and aloe vera are natural remedies that can help with the discomfort.

Going to the bathroom after childbirth may seem scary. Urine stings as it hits the raw skin. Having a bowel movement feels like you are going to split your skin or stiches open. A few tricks: fill a water bottle with warm water. As you urinate, squirt yourself with the water to rinse the urine from the skin immediately. Also, take stool softeners, increase your fiber intake, and drink prune juice to prevent constipation.

Stress and Urge Incontinence

During the first year after childbirth, half of women have urinary incontinence and 17 percent have fecal incontinence. One third of these will remain incontinent for many years to come. Some women lose urine occasionally, when they cough or laugh. Others leak during sex, walking up the stairs, or when they pick up their baby. Unfortunately, there is no quick fix for this problem, and many women learn to put up with it for a lifetime. They find themselves scouting out the nearest bathroom, wearing pads, and limiting how much fluid they drink. Although most new moms are willing to live with these symptoms while they are busy with a new baby, they don't want to deal with it forever.

The muscles of the pelvic floor, which support the bladder like a sling, also control urination. Pregnancy and childbirth weaken these muscles and damage the muscles or nerves so that urine comes out involuntarily. In some cases, the muscles completely detach from the pubic bone. Overall, 15 percent of women with a vaginal delivery sustain an injury to the pelvic floor that doesn't heal for years. Women who push for a long time have the highest risk of incontinence, but pregnancy itself can weaken the muscles. Having a cesarean doesn't prevent this problem. After a vaginal birth, 50 percent of women will leak urine, and after a cesarean, 23 percent will.

Limiting damage to the pelvic floor from pregnancy and childbirth is nearly impossible. Therefore, the focus should be on how to repair it. Kegel exercises are the most commonly prescribed treatment, but they only strengthen the muscles themselves. They can't reattach the muscle to the bone or heal a nerve injury. Kegel exercises during pregnancy do not decrease the risk of incontinence. Many women begin Kegels right after birth. However, some experts suggest that the injury to the pelvic floor should be treated like any other sports injury. If you strain a muscle playing a sport, you rest it for four to six weeks so it can heal prior to rehabilitation. Then the strengthening exercises can begin. Further research is needed to know which approach is best.

How to perform Kegels: The easiest way to learn how to exercise these muscles is to stop your urine midstream. The muscle that you feel contracting is part of your pelvic floor. You should contract the muscle for three seconds, then release it for three seconds. Repeat this ten times per day.

Although incontinence is common after birth, it shouldn't be considered normal. If it interferes with your lifestyle, limits what you like to do, or makes you self-conscious, you should try to repair it. If Kegels haven't helped, a physical therapist who specializes in the pelvic floor can be invaluable. Some insurance plans will cover this type of therapy. Surgery is also available to lift the bladder back to its normal location.

Weight Loss

How do the celebrities do it? They have a baby and are on the red carpet six weeks later without an ounce of baby weight in sight. The baby, placenta, and amniotic fluid account for 13 pounds that are immediately lost after delivery. You can expect to lose half of the weight by six weeks postpartum and the rest over the next five to six months. Keep in mind that celebrities, of course, have access to private chefs and trainers who prepare healthy meals and get them in the gym for a few hours every day.

Pregnancy is a major risk factor for becoming overweight or obese. One year after birth, most women are heavier than before they became pregnant. In fact, one third of normal-weight women become overweight or obese after having a baby. Much of the difficulty losing weight occurs because over half of women gain more weight than is recommended.

While it would seem logical that the extra calories needed to produce breast milk—about 500 calories per day—would help with weight loss, many studies show that the average amount lost is essentially the same for women who are nursing and those who aren't. This may be because many women don't breastfeed exclusively, so the calories needed to produce milk amount to less than 500 per day. In addition, the hormone prolactin acts as an appetite stimulant, making breastfeeding women feel hungry and eat more.

Belly bands and abdominal binders will not help you lose weight; they only help with posture and back support, holding things in place as a girdle or corset would do. While they may help you fit into your old clothes, they don't make the extra pounds come off any faster.

Strategies for Losing Weight

- Don't gain an excessive amount during the pregnancy.
- Treat exercise like an appointment you cannot break.
- Plan meals so you don't find yourself eating whatever happens to be in the refrigerator.
- Take a walk every day with the baby—even if it's just for 15 to 20 minutes.
- Stock up on healthy foods that don't require preparation—yogurt, prepackaged sliced fruit, cereal, and salads.

You and Your Partner, Postpartum

A baby can bring great joy to its parents, but there is no doubt that having an infant impacts all members of the household—particularly the mother and her partner.

Your Relationship

Your relationship with your partner will undoubtedly change when you bring home a baby. Adding a baby to your family can be a bond to bring you closer, but also can make life more complicated and exacerbate any preexisting issues. A recent survey showed that 90 percent of couples say they feel more tension, 60 percent feel less satisfied in their marriage, and 15 percent of fathers leave the relationship within one year of birth.

After delivery, a mother's primary focus is her baby. Her partner may feel left out, overwhelmed by responsibilities, or unsure of what is expected of him. Lack of sleep and time for intimacy can create a distance between partners. A new mom gets lots of physical contact during the day from her baby, especially if she is nursing. When it is time for bed, she simply wants to sleep and would rather have some space of her own without being touched. Her need for physical space can make her partner feel rejected, which can ultimately lead to resentment.

Communicating your needs and feelings is critical to keeping your relationship strong during this challenging time. Even before the baby is born, you can discuss the expected duties and responsibilities of each partner. You can plan financially so that stress is kept to a minimum. Emotional intimacy can be achieved by doing something nice for each other, being considerate of one's needs, being supportive of life goals, and not putting each other down. If you do not know how to foster emotional intimacy, all you need to do is ask your partner: What would light you up? What can I do to make your life better? You may need to be the one to initiate intimacy. You can do something nice for him that may inspire him to reciprocate. A simple approach is always to speak to each other in a loving way.

Sexual Function

Postpartum sexual dysfunction is very common in new families. Most issues revolve around a lack of desire for sex and pain during intercourse. Fatigue due to lack of sleep and the stress of taking care of a new baby makes sex the last thing on many women's mind. Women may also feel uncomfortable with the physical changes in their body and want to avoid intimate contact.

Discomfort from healing vaginal lacerations or episiotomies also deters sexual activity. Breastfeeding lowers estrogen levels, so the vaginal tissue becomes dry and loses its stretchiness, similar to what post-menopausal women feel. In one quarter of women, painful intercourse persists for years.

Most women have resumed sexual activity by three months postpartum. Medically, intercourse can be resumed as early as two weeks after delivery as long as the perineum is healed. However, most women are not ready for sex this soon, even if it doesn't involve penetration.

Fertility in the Postpartum

Women who are not breastfeeding will start ovulating six to eight weeks postpartum. Women who nurse may not ovulate at all during breastfeeding. However, they may release an egg unexpectedly and become pregnant. If you don't want to become pregnant, you should use a contraceptive, whether you are nursing or not.

Managing as a New Mom

Sometimes a new mom can't catch a break. It seems no matter what you do, someone will have an opinion about why you shouldn't be doing it or how you are doing it wrong. Everything is under scrutiny, from nursing too long, to being a stay at home mom, to working too much. If you chose an elective cesarean, you may be judged. If you chose a home birth, someone will find fault in it. People are going to have opinions and share them freely. Don't let them get to you. If you have done your research and made your choices, stick to your guns and let any attempts at shaming roll off your back.

Managing at Home with Your New Baby

- Accept help: If someone offers to bring you dinner or help do the laundry, say yes. Extended family is great for doing things you don't have time to do.

- Try to get one hour per day by yourself: After nursing, ask your partner or mother to watch the baby so you can have some time to yourself. Take a warm bath. Watch some mindless TV. Get caught up on emails. Do anything that doesn't involve the baby.
- Go outside every day—even if it is just for 15 minutes: Take a short walk with the baby or sit outdoors. The fresh air does wonders when you spend nearly all day inside.
- Sleep when the baby sleeps: Of course, this is easier said than done at first. It is hard to fall asleep during the day at the drop of a hat. If you cannot sleep, close your eyes and lie down while listening to some soft music. Even this time of relaxation can be rejuvenating.
- Don't feel bad about asking visitors to leave: Family and friends may not know the best way to help you. They want to play with the baby while you are trying to learn how to nurse. It's okay to redirect them to assist you with some chores or even ask them to leave while you concentrate on the baby alone.

the doctor's diary

For many hours of labor, as well as the nine months that have preceded it, the mom-to-be is the center of attention. She is asked how she is feeling, does she want some water, or does she want a blanket. During the second stage of labor when she is pushing—all eyes are on her, everyone is giving support and words of encouragement, and taking care of her by wiping her forehead, or giving her ice chips between contractions. With her cheering section on hand, the baby is finally out. She holds her newborn for a minute or two. Then it is whisked away to the warmer in the room to be dried and suctioned. The crowd in the room turns to the warmer and stands around it in awe. The nurse is listening to the baby's heart and lungs; the new dad, grandma, and aunt watch happily. The new mother is left alone, just with me, as I check for any tears or excessive bleeding. She tries to peer around the bodies to see her baby. As I am repairing her tear, I glance up. Sometimes I see a look of relief and contentment, but other times I see that she seems to be wondering, "What about me?" In just a second, the baby has become the center of attention. The shift is palpable.

At the postpartum visit, I always inquire about how my patients are feeling, and how they are coping with the sleepless nights and the stresses of nursing. Most moms tell me it's been rough, a lot harder than they expected. Nothing could have prepared them for this. They tell me that they've been disappointed in their partners, that their partners aren't as helpful as they expected or hoped. They confess that their postpartum support mostly comes from three a.m. Internet searches. They feel bad that they haven't been able to do everything themselves—taking care of the baby, keeping the house clean, and cooking meals.

Babies are born every day. So, women assume they should be able to hit the ground running. But my patients don't see themselves as someone who is recuperating. They are not "sick." Instead, they think they should be supermoms. This attitude is engrained in American culture. In fact, the United States is the only industrialized nation that doesn't have mandatory paid maternity leave. The postpartum rituals of being cared for by family and friends, of eating certain foods, or of staying home have been replaced by the rush to get back to work—or back to taking care of everything in the home including the new baby. In other cultures, the "forty days" of rest is still observed while in the United States, the pressure to do it all is overwhelming. I try to encourage my patients to take care of themselves. Only then can they be good mothers.

Every once in a while, I have a mom who is able to look past the pressure and anxiety to recognize just how special this time is. I remember one mom who told me her favorite time was the middle of the night, when the house was quiet. Her husband and other daughter were sleeping. She said that she enjoyed that time in the room lit by a nightlight when she could hold her baby against her body and smell the top of her head while the baby nursed. As exhausted as she was, these quiet, undisturbed moments made it all worth it.

SOLUTIONS FOR A BETTER BIRTH EXPERIENCE

Our childbirth system isn't perfect. Some would even say it's in a crisis. Doctors and midwives, hospitals, insurance companies, lawmakers, and mothers need to work together to improve the experience for everyone. As someone who has helped many women bring their children into the world, I have a number of ideas that I think would benefit mothers and babies during this most significant life event.

What Mothers Can Do

- Seek a birthing environment that allows your baby to stay with you after delivery and promotes the "golden hour." By avoiding hospitals that do not support this, hospitals will be forced to change their protocols.
- Open a dialogue with your provider about what you and your family hope for during your birth by preparing a

birth plan. Having this conversation forces providers to think about the justification of their rules. In the past, women received an enema and had their pubic hair shaved when they came to the hospital. Low-risk childbirth took place in sterile operating rooms. Episiotomies were common. By challenging these routine procedures, women have forced the medical community to evaluate their benefits and risks, and to conclude that many of these otherwise routine actions weren't necessary. The same can happen with practices like requiring women to stay in bed during labor, to have an IV or continuous fetal monitoring, and to undergo cesareans without a strong medical indication.

- Call your insurance company to demand coverage for midwives and birthing centers.
- Be aware of the ramifications of testing. If you prefer to see an obstetrician at every prenatal visit and choose to have all possible testing, you are more likely to undergo medical interventions during delivery. By changing your expectations, you may be able to avoid doing things that aren't necessary.
- Know that you can change providers. If you find that your provider doesn't answer your questions or spends very little time with you during your appointments, you should switch providers. If a physician loses patients, she may reconsider her bedside manner and office practices.
- Be supportive. We need to be supportive of each other's decisions about childbirth. For some, labor is empowering. For others, using an epidural and blocking the pain feels right. Stereotyping and putting people down because of their decisions never changes minds and only creates animosity.

What Doctors Can Do

- Make their cesarean and induction rates public. This allows patients to choose a provider who supports their goals and encourages doctors to keep their rates at reasonable levels.
- Be trained in breech deliveries and the vaginal delivery of twins and breech babies.
- Encourage women to have a vaginal birth after cesarean (VBAC).
- Stop overtreating the natural experience. There is no doubt that modern medicine has saved numerous lives of mothers and babies but procedures intended for high-risk pregnancies shouldn't be extended to all low-risk mothers.
- Recognize that not all interventions lead to better outcomes.
- Do not prioritize convenience over the best outcome for the patient.
- Examine the necessity of routine practices, such as IVs in labor and suctioning of newborns at birth, and change practice patterns accordingly.
- Only recommend interventions that have been scientifically proven to give better outcomes.
- Collaborate with midwives in the community in a positive and respectful way.
- Teach their patients that their body is designed for birth so that women can feel confident that they will be successful.

What Midwives Can Do

- Insist on rigorous, uniform training and testing so they are equipped to deal with any emergent situation.
- Work with lawmakers to make licensing available in all states.

- Limit their practice to low-risk pregnancies and transfer patients when complications arise. As much as a midwife would like to help her patient achieve the birth she desires, she needs to remain realistic about the scope of her practice.
- Improve safety protocols. To improve home birth safety, midwives should be required to have an agreement with a physician, carry malpractice insurance, and report their outcomes to the public.

What Hospitals Can Do

- Provide better postpartum care that is quiet and unobtrusive with skin-to-skin contact for mothers and babies.
- Change the model of care on the labor and delivery unit to include more laborists and midwives who can deliver patients without the pressure of a tight schedule, thereby reducing the cesarean rates.
- Make cesarean and induction rates at the hospital public.
- Support the natural cesarean.
- Adopt policies and procedures that are evidence-based, not liability-based.
- Create an environment that mimics being at home by building birthing centers within or adjacent to hospitals.
- Be required to train staff how to accommodate home birth transfers in a respectful way.
- Have lactation consultants on staff and remove gift bags of formula from postpartum rooms.

What Lawmakers Can Do

- In every state, address the issue of licensing midwives. With clear training requirements, testing, and accreditation, patients can be assured that the provider they choose is qualified to care for them. When midwives are licensed, they are more easily integrated into the general health system. Physicians will be able to partner with licensed midwives so that patients can seamlessly transfer care in case of an emergency.

- Create legislation limiting high-risk deliveries in the home that will ultimately make home birth safer.
- As in many countries around the world, the United States should provide mandatory paid maternity leave so new mothers can have time to take care of their babies with less financial stress. Postpartum services at home should also be an option, such as a nurse or lactation consultant who can visit patients in the first few weeks after delivery.
- Do your part to reform malpractice laws. Caps on malpractice settlements will discourage attorneys from accepting cases that don't have merit.

What Insurance Companies Can Do

- Cover the cost of hiring a doula. By doing so, insurers will save money in the long run, as the use of doulas decreases preterm deliveries and cesareans.
- Cover the cost of licensed midwives and birthing centers.

Improving obstetrical care in the United States should be a goal for all involved. I believe that if women, doctors, midwives, hospitals, the legal profession, and insurance companies take a close look at how they view a woman's health and well-being during delivery, we can give women the birth experience they desire efficiently, safely, and happily.

RESOURCES

Websites

American Academy of Pediatrics
www.aap.org

American Board of Obstetrics and Gynecology
www.abog.org

American College of Nurse-Midwives
www.midwife.org

American College of Obstetricians and Gynecologists
www.acog.org

Be the Match Registry
www.bethematch.org

Childbirth and Postpartum Professional Association
www.cappa.net

Consortium on Safe Labor
https://csl.nichd.nih.gov/

DONA International
www.dona.org

Environmental Working Group's Skin Deep Cosmetic Safety Database
www.ewg.org/skindeep

International Board of Lactation Consultant Examiners (IBLCE)
www.iblce.org

The Leapfrog Group
www.leapfroggroup.org/compare-hospitals

Midwives Alliance of North America
www.mana.org

North American Registry of Midwives
www.narm.org

Society for Maternal-Fetal Medicine
www.smfm.org

NOTES

Chapter 1: What Does a "Natural" Birth Mean, Anyway?

1. P. M. Dunn, "Louise Bourgeois (1563–1636): Royal Midwife of France" in *Archives of Diseases in Childhood—Fetal & Neonatal Edition* 89, no. 2, BJM Publishing Group & Royal College of Paediatrics and Child Health, 2004, http://fn.bmj.com/content/89/2/F185.full.

Chapter 3: Natural Choices

1. L. Glynn et al., "When Stress Happens Matters: Effects of Earthquake Timing on Stress Responsivity in Pregnancy," *American Journal of Obstetrics & Gynecology* 184, no. 4 (2001): 637–42.

2. E. Davis and C. Sandman, "Prenatal Psychobiological Predictors of Anxiety Risk in Preadolescent Children," *Psychoneuroendocrinology* 37, no. 8 (August 2012): 1224–33.

3. S. Entringer and P. Wadhua, "Prenatal Stress and Developmental Programming of Human Health and Disease Risk," *Current Opinion in Endocrinology, Diabetes, and Obesity* 17, no. 6 (December 2010): 507–16.

4. C. Hobel et al., "The West Los Angeles Preterm Birth Prevention Project," *American Journal of Obstetrics and Gynecology* 170, no. 1 (January 1994): 54–62.

5. J. Reefhuis et al., "Specific SSRIs and Birth Defects," *British Medical Journal* 351 (2015): h3190.

6. A. Aris and S. Leblanc, "Maternal and Fetal Exposure to Pesticides Associated to Genetically Modified Foods in Eastern Townships of Quebec," *Reproductive Toxicology* 21, no. 4 (2011): 528–33.

7. A. Frazier et al., "Prospective Study of Peripregnancy Consumption of Peanuts or Tree Nuts by Mothers and the Risk of Peanut or Tree Nut Allergy in Their Offspring," *Journal of the American Medical Association Pediatrics* 168, no. 2 (2013): 156–62.

8. K. Evenson and F. Wen, "National Trends in Self-reported Physical Activity and Sedentary Behaviors Among Pregnant Women," *Preventive Medicine* 50 (2010): 123–28.

9. See http://www.babycenter.com/0_folic-acid-why-you-need-it-before -and-during-pregnancy_476.bc?page=2; http://www.mthfrsupport.com .au/wp-content/uploads/2014/04/Avoid-Folic-Acid-Containg-Foods-and -Drugs-National.pdf.

10. T. Chaban and R. Tannock, "Environmental Factors in ADHD," AboutKidsHealth, last modified November 30, 2009, http://www.about kidshealth.ca/en/resourcecentres/adhd/aboutadhd/whatcausesadhd /pages/environmental-factors-in-adhd.aspx.

11. S. Swan et al., "Prenatal Phthalate Exposure and Reduced Masculine Play in Boys," *International Journal of Andrology* 33, no. 2 (2010): 259–69.

12. T. Woodruff, A. Zota, and J. Schwartz, "Environmental Chemicals in Pregnant Women in the United States," *Environmental Health Perspectives* 119, no. 6 (June 2011): 878–85.

13. Reefhuis et al., "Specific SSRIs and Birth Defects."

Chapter 4: Choosing Who, Where, and How

1. E. Hodnett et al., "Continuous Support for Women During Childbirth," Cochrane Database of Systemic Reviews, no. 7, article number CD003766 (2013).

2. K. Kozhimannil et al., "Modeling the Cost-effectiveness of Doula Care Associated with Reductions in Preterm Birth and Cesarean Delivery," *Birth* 43, no. 1 (2016): 20–27.

3. S. Stapleton, C. Osborne, and J. Illuzzi, "Outcome of Care in Birth Centers: Demonstration of a Durable Model," *Journal of Midwifery and Women's Health* 58, no. 1 (2013): 3–14.

4. P. Brocklehurst et al., "Perinatal and Maternal Outcome by Planned Place of Birth for Healthy Women with Low Risk Pregnancies," *British Medical Journal* 343 (2011): d7400.

5. A. De Jonge et al., "Perinatal Mortality and Morbidity up to 28 Days After Low-Risk Planned Home Birth," *British Journal of Obstetrics and Gynaecology* 122 (2015): 720–28.

6. M. Cheyney et al., "Outcomes of Care for 16,924 Planned Home-births in the United States," *Journal of Midwifery and Women's Health* 59 (2014): 17–27.

7. J. Wax et al., "Maternal and Newborn Outcomes in Planned Home Birth Versus Planned Hospital Births," *American Journal of Obstetrics & Gynecology* 203 (2010): 243e1–e8.

8. OHA (Oregon Health Authority), Public Health Division, "Preliminary Data on Oregon Birth Outcomes, by Planned Birth Place and Attendant," Pursuant to: HB 2380 (2011), 2013, https://olis.leg.state.or.us/liz/2013R1/Downloads/CommitteeMeetingDocument/10024.

9. J. Wax, M. Pinette, and A. Cartin, "Home Versus Hospital Birth—Process and Outcomes," *Obstetrical and Gynecological Survey* 65 (2010): 132–40.

10. F. Chervenak et al., "Home birth: The Obstetrician's Ethical Response," *Contemporary OBGYN* 60, no. 7 (July 2015): 44–48.

Chapter 5: Is This Test or Intervention Necessary?

1. E. Declercq et al., "Listening to Mothers III: New Mothers Speak Out. Report of the Third National U.S. Survey of Women's Childbearing Experiences," New York: Childbirth Connection, June 2013.

2. L. Bricker, N. Medley, and J. Pratt, "Routine Ultrasound in Late Pregnancy," Cochrane Database (2015): 6 Art CD001451.

3. T. Stacey et al., "Maternal Perception of Fetal Activity and Late Stillbirth Risk," *Birth* 38, no. 4 (December 2011): 311–16.

4. C. McCall, D. Grime, and A. Lyerly, "'Therapeutic' Bed Rest in Pregnancy: Unethical and Unsupported by Data," *Obstetrics and Gynecology* 121, no. 6 (2013): 1305–8.

Chapter 6: Expecting the Unexpected

1. M. Coyle, C. Smith, and B. Peat, "Cephalic Version by Moxibustion for Breech Presentation," Cochrane Database (2012), article number CD003928.

2. K. Grootscholten et al., "External Cephalic Version-Related Risks: A Meta-analysis," *Obstetrics and Gynecology* 112, no. 5 (2008): 1143–51.

3. J. Hemelaar, L. Lim, and L. Impey, "The Impact of an ECV Service Is Limited by Antenatal Breech Detection," *Birth* 42, no. 2 (June 2015): 165–72.

4. M. Cheyney et al., "Outcomes of Care for 16,924 Planned Home Births in the United States," *Journal of Midwifery and Women's Health* 59, no. 1 (2014): 17–27.

5. M. Hannah et al., "Planned Cesarean Section Versus Planned Vaginal Birth for Breech Presentation at Term," *Lancet* 356 (October 2000): 1375–83.

6. J. Dempsey et al., "Prospective Study of Gestational Diabetes Mellitus Risk in Relation to Maternal Recreational Physical Activity Before and During Pregnancy," *American Journal of Epidemiology* 159, no. 7 (April 1, 2004): 663–70.

7. S. Gabbe, J. Niebyl, and J. Simpson, *Obstetrics: Normal and Problem Pregnancies*, 5th ed. (Philadelphia: Churchill Livingstone Elsevier, 2007): 836–37.

8. A. Jukic et al., "Length of Human Pregnancy and Contributors to its Natural Variation," *Human Reproduction* 28, no. 10 (2013): 2848–55.

9. E. Declercq et al., "Listening to Mothers III: New Mothers Speak Out. Report of the Third National U.S. Survey of Women's Childbearing Experiences," New York: Childbirth Connection, June 2013.

10. A. Wallis et al., "Secular Trends in the Rates of Preeclampsia, Eclampsia and Gestational Hypertension, United States 1987–2004," *American Journal of Hypertension* 21 (2008): 521–26.

11. A. Klebanoff et al., "Fish Consumption, Erythrocyte Fatty Acids, and Preterm Birth," *Obstetrics and Gynecology* 117, no. 5 (May 2011): 1071–77.

12. W. Grobman et al., "Activity Restriction Among Women with a Short Cervix," *Obstetrics and Gynecology* 121, no. 6 (June 2013): 1181–86.

13. J. Bardos et al., "A National Survey on Public Perceptions of Miscarriage," *Obstetrics and Gynecology* 125, no. 6 (2015): 1313–20.

14. J. Barrett et al., "A Randomized Trial of Planned Cesarean or Vaginal Delivery for Twin Pregnancy," *New England Journal of Medicine* 369 (2013): 1295–1305, doi: 10.1056/NEJMoa1214939.

Chapter 7: What You Need to Know, and Need to Ask, About Labor

1. B. Nesheim and R. Kinge, "Performance of Acupuncture as Labor Analgesia in the Clinical Setting," *Acta Obstetricia et Gynecologica Scandinavica* 85 no. 4 (2006): 441–43.

2. K. Madden et al., "Hypnosis for Pain Management During Labor and Childbirth," Cochrane Database 19, no. 5 (May 2016): CD 009356.

3. B. Trolle et al., "The Effect of Sterile Water Blocks on Low Back Labor Pain," *American Journal of Obstetrics & Gynecology* 164 (1991): 1277–81.

4. T. Field, "Pregnancy and Labor Massage," *Expert Review of Obstetrics & Gynecology* 5, no. 2 (March 2010): 177–81.

5. M. Bovbjerg, M. Cheyney and C. Everson, "Maternal and Newborn Outcomes Following Waterbirth," *Journal of Midwifery and Women's Health* 61, no 1 (January 2016): 11–20.

6. M. Odent, "Is Participation of the Father at Birth Dangerous?" *Midwifery Today* 1999 (1999): 23–24.

7. K. Lien, J. DeLancey, and J. Ashton-Miller, "Biomechanical Analyses of the Efficacy of Maternal Effort on Second-Stage Progress," *Obstetrics and Gynecology* 113, no. 4 (2009): 873–80.

8. J. Golay, S. Vedam, and L. Sorger, "The Squatting Position and the Second Stage of Labor," *Birth* 20, no. 2 (1993): 73–78.

9. "Cord Blood Banking for Future Transplantation," American Academy of Pediatrics Policy Statement, *Pediatrics* 119 (2007): 165.

Chapter 8: Interventions in the Delivery Room: Exception or Rule?

1. E. Declercq et al., "Listening to Mothers III: New Mothers Speak Out. Report of the Third National U.S. Survey of Women's Childbearing Experiences," New York: Childbirth Connection, June 2013.

2. G. Molina et al., "Relationship Between Cesarean Delivery Rate and Maternal and Neonatal Mortality," *Journal of the American Medical Association* 314, no. 21 (2015): 2263–70.

3. M. Dominguez-Bello et al., "Partial Restoration of the Microbiota of Cesarean-born Infants via Vaginal Microbial Transfer," *Nature Medicine* 2 (2016): 250–53.

4. E. Prior et al., "Breastfeeding After Cesarean Delivery," *American Journal of Clinical Nutrition* 95, no. 5 (May 2012): 1113–35.

5. S. Gabbe and G. Holzman, "Obstetricians' Choice of Delivery," *Lancet* 357 (2001): 722.

6. S. Tracy et al., "Birth Outcomes Associated with Interventions in Labor Amongst Low Risk Women," *Women and Birth* 20, no. 2 (2007): 41–48.

7. R. Smyth, C. Markham, and T. Dowswell, "Amniotomy for Shortening Spontaneous Labor," Cochrane Database (2013), article number CD006167.

8. C. Mendelson et al., "The Aspiration of Stomach Contents into the Lungs During Obstetric Anesthesia," *American Journal of Obstetrics & Gynecology* 52 (1946): 191–205.

9. P. Nielsen et al., "Intra- and Inter-Observer Variability in the Assessment of Intrapartum Cardiotocograms. *Acta Obstetricia Gynecologica Scandinavica* 66 (1987): 421–24.

10. K. Cox et al., "Planned Home VBAC in the United States, 2004–2009," *Birth* 42, no. 4 (2015): 299–308.

Chapter 9: The Unpredictable, Wonderful, Very Special Day

1. M. Hannah et al., "Induction of Labor Compared with Expectant Management for Prelabor Rupture of Membranes at Term," *New England Journal of Medicine* 334 (1996): 1005–10.

2. J. Morris et al., "Immediate Delivery Compared with Expectant Management After Preterm Prelabor Rupture of Membranes Close to Term," *Lancet* 387 (2016): 444–52.

Chapter 10: After Delivery

1. I. G. Wickes, "A History of Infant Feeding, Part I," *Archives of Disease in Childhood* 28 (1953a): 151–58.

2. C. Colen and D. Ramey, "Is Breast Truly Best? Estimating the Effects of Breastfeeding on Long-term Child Health and Wellbeing in the United States Using Sibling Comparisons," *Social Science and Medicine* 109 (2014): 55–65.

3. B. Gibbs et al., "Breastfeeding, Parenting and Early Cognitive Development," *Journal of Pediatrics* 14, no. 3 (2014): 487.

4. K. Kabir, J. Sheeder, and S. Kelly, "Identifying Postpartum Depression: Are Three Questions as Good as Ten?" *Journal of Pediatrics* 122 (2008): e696-e702.

INDEX